Supersex: Your Guide to Lifelong Loving

**Published by
Sunday Books
London**

in association with
**Peter Grose Ltd
Monmouth**

Cover picture: Mark Lawrence
Photography by: Mark Lawrence, Harry Ormesher, Ian Spratt

British Library C.I.P.
A catalogue record for this book is available from the British Library.

ISBN: 1-898-88504-4

Supersex: Your Guide to Lifelong Loving

by
Roslyn Grose

**Sunday
Books**

London

Acknowledgements

Thank you to all the people—experts, friends and strangers—who have provided the information that follows. In particular, thanks to:

RELATE (Herbert Gray College, Little Church Street, Rugby, Warwickshire CV21 3AP), whose spokespeople, counsellors and sex therapists have always been so willing to share their knowledge.

THE FAMILY PLANNING ASSOCIATION (27 Mortimer Street, London W1N 7RJ), whose excellent publications cannot be bettered for the quality and clarity of their information.

ISSUE (The National Fertility Association, 509 Aldridge Road, Great Barr, Birmingham B44 8NA), for fertility facts and advice.

Contents

1. SUPERSEX: *What is it?*   3

2. SEX MYTHS: *Who told you that!*   7

3. LOVE AND ATTRACTION: *Magic—or can you turn it on?*   13

4. COME-ONS: *Can it hurt to flirt?*   21

5. BODYTALK: *How we move from date to mate*   29

6. THE GEOGRAPHY OF LOVE: *Chart your way to ecstasy*   37

7. THE FIRST TIME : *Starting a new relationship*   45

8. FOREPLAY: *Love that lasts all day*   53

9. THE POSITION IS THIS: *Sexual positions—a consumer guide*   61

10. WHERE TO DO IT: *Bedrooms, bike sheds and back seats*   71

11. SEX DRIVE: *The Owner's Manual*   81

12. ORGASM: *Making the earth move—is that it?*   87

13. THE BIG OH-NO! *Your mate wants something and you don't*   93

14. FANTASY SEX: *How real can you get!*   101

15. BEDTIME MANNERS: *Animal passion is OK, but don't be a pig*   113

16. HOLIDAY SEX: *When the lovin' is easy*   117

17. CONTRACEPTION: *The pros and condoms*   123

18. MAKING BABIES: *How easy is it?*   129

19. PROBLEMS: *Too tired? Too busy? Too nervous?*   135

20. WHEN KIDS ARRIVE: *Sex after parenthood*   147

Supersex: Your Guide to Lifelong Loving

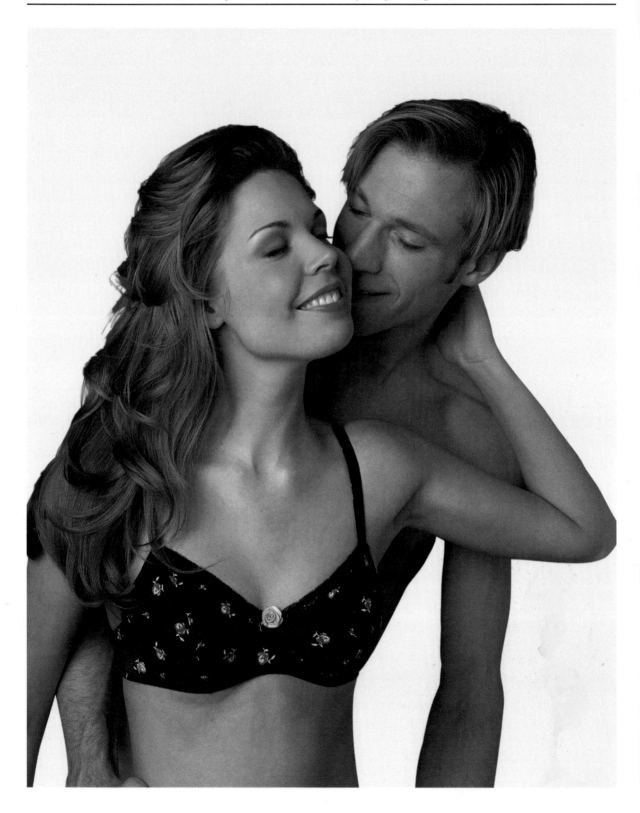

SUPERSEX

What is it?

It's hard to remember the first inkling you had of sex. Was it when your parents mysteriously shut their bedroom door in your face and ignored your four-year-old kicks and shouts? Was it when they shuffled about looking shifty when you asked what 'blowjob' meant as you pored over the Sunday newspapers, grappling to work out what was going on in the stories beside pictures of grown-ups in their underwear?

It may have been when you went home from school and told mum and dad the terrific story you heard in the playground about the gorilla and the banana: after they'd choked on their tea they'd asked a lot of questions about who told you and what other stories were going the rounds of the local Infants and Juniors.

You might have seen words on walls or heard them whispered by classmates who claimed to know what they meant. Their explanations left you none the wiser, just plagued with new worries to set your imagination rioting out of control.

From those first wonderings about something that seemed to be THE secret of life, you probably blundered through a maze of misinformation from which many adults still struggle to emerge clear-headed.

Once roused, sexual curiosity can last a lifetime. Possibly the most exciting thing about sex is that you can't know it all. Yet there are couples all over the country who claim to be dying of sexual boredom—if you're an advice-column addict like me, you'll know that bed-and-bored is one of the perennials of the complaints charts.

Could this be due to some people's sexual knowledge not extending beyond the biology? They know which part of the male anatomy slots into which part of the female; how sperm from the male swim up into the female's uterus, like a shoal of racing tadpoles, and fertilise any egg they can find. They know it's supposed to be fun but they don't really understand what all the fuss is about. Could they be missing some vital part of the exercise—or have they simply been pounding the mattress with the wrong mate?

It would not be human not to speculate about what others do behind closed bedroom doors or indeed in the back seats of cars, in quiet corners of parks or in dark corners of discos. Nor would it be surprising if we sometimes suspected that others were making the earth tremble every night while we were registering minus-nothing on the Richter scale.

Despite the zillions of words written and spoken on the subject, the books, magazines, films and videos, there are still aspects of sex we don't know about, haven't experienced or find puzzling, worrying or even disgusting.

What's normal? That's the unanswerable question. Experts of various kinds have endlessly probed our sexual habits in the effort to find out. Their conclusion is al-

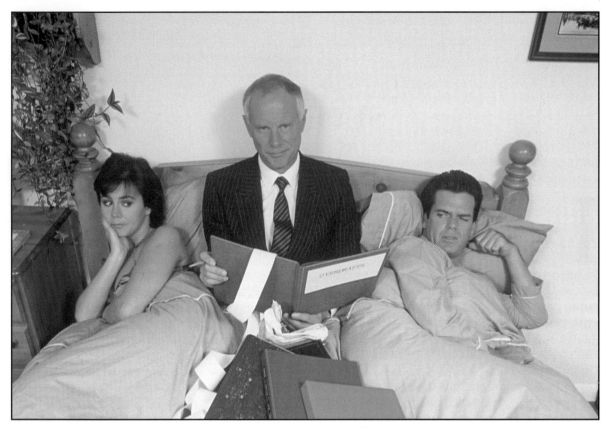

Most GPs are hard-pressed enough dealing with the ill and injured without having to give sex lessons.

ways that with sex there is no such thing as normal. Virtually anything you do of a sexual nature is acceptable as long as you're not forcing someone else to do something they don't want to do. Normal is five-times-a-night sex if that's what you're used to—or twice a year, if that keeps you satisfied.

But as for what everyone else does, how often, where and when—how do you find out, when it's such a private activity? Most people don't want to reveal the details of their sex lives—and those who do tend to exaggerate, embroider or otherwise distort the truth.

Secrecy, lies, exaggeration—it's a wonder the human race isn't threatened with extinction due to our befuddling of the facts of life.

No small part of the problem, at least in Britain, is that we cannot agree on who should tell us where babies come from, the difference between a blowjob and a blow-dry and what to do at a Mars bar party. Parents get stammery with embarrassment as soon as a child fires a facts-of-life question at them. Dad and mum pass the buck between themselves until kids realise they're better off asking their peers: the answers might be a bit dodgy but at least they'll get answers.

Teachers seem to be less embarrassed about offering sex education. But they are frequently attacked for their efforts by agitated parents who claim not to approve of what their kids are being taught.

Doctors are often held up as the most reliable source of sex information. But sex is not a disease and most GPs are hard-pressed enough dealing with the ill and injured without having to give sex lessons. Besides, talking sex with a patient of the opposite gender could possibly be hazardous these days when it might be claimed afterwards to be sexual harrassment. And anyway, many doctors are about as qualified to give sex guidance as to offer tennis coaching.

So who's an expert, then? Sex therapists and marriage counsellors can be a great help if your sex life is in trouble. But what most of us need is not a repair job. We just want reassurance that the neighbours aren't in on some magical sexual secret that's so far been kept from us. We'd like to be sexually informed, if not necessarily experienced in every erotic art. We seek a guideline here, a pleasure boost there, some fresh ideas to tickle ours and our partner's fancy.

What most of us would like to know is, are we are having the most fun we could possibly enjoy with our chosen lover?

As a journalist, I started talking to people about their sex lives in the early Seventies—both men and women, friends and strangers—and have never stopped. Hundreds have spilled their intimate secrets, wanting to share their experiences and to know that others were having similar joys, doubts, wonders and worries. Most were people with no really serious problems, wanting to talk to someone who wasn't their spouse, their next-door-neighbour, their parent, close friend or workmate—an impartial outsider they could use as a sounding board. Along the way I also talked to psychologists, psychiatrists, sex therapists, counsellors, GPs, the occasional anthropologist and zoologist, anyone who'd done any serious study in the sex field.

What makes sex fun? And how can I get maximum pleasure from it? These are the questions I would have liked to ask my own mother but somehow didn't think of it at the time. She tried, at one stage, to begin my sex education by giving me a booklet on reproduction with a lot of detail about the mating habits of frogs. The back section, dealing with humans, was pinned together with a safety pin and she gave strict instructions not to read it. But the bit about the frogs was of so little interest, and so puzzling, I had no urge to read further. That pin stayed in place, for all I know, till it rusted. There ended mum's sex lessons.

So the rest of the world has had to fill me in on what she forgot to mention—thank you everyone. I've unpinned the following pages for those who want more fun in their sex life, more info about what others do and more answers to questions they're too embarrassed to ask. And promise not to talk about frogs.

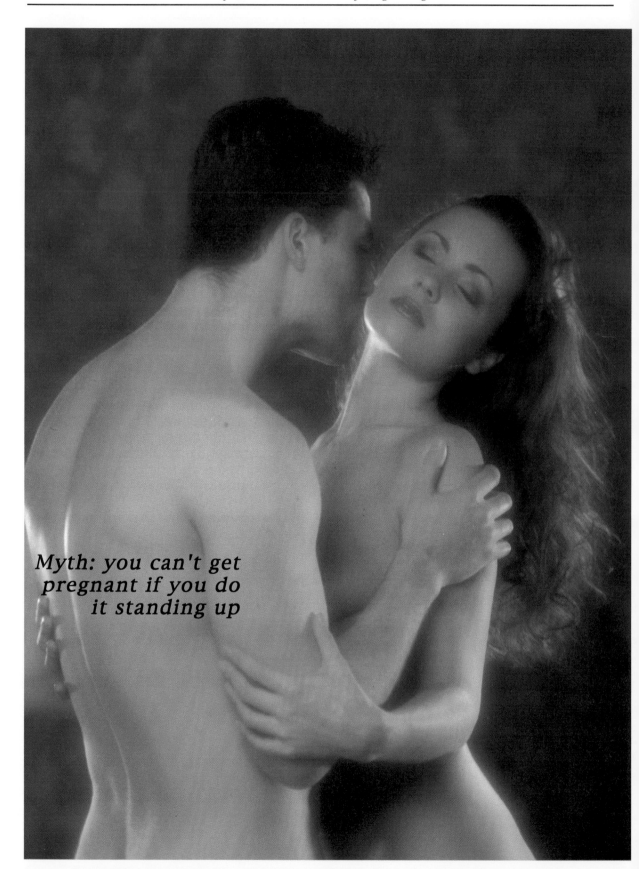

Myth: you can't get pregnant if you do it standing up

SEX MYTHS
Who told you that?

The secrecy and mystery that so often surround sex have produced so many myths, half-truths, lies, legends and fantasies that it can be hard to sort fact from fiction.

Here are some of the most widespread barmy beliefs—and the True Facts to set the record straight.

You can't get pregnant if you have sex standing up.

Just testing—no one really believes that one any more, do they? They do? Some people obviously have a problem with gravity here, believing that what goes up must come down. That is, the sperm that shoots into the vagina at the vital moment of the sex act will fall out immediately after and not swim about looking for an egg to fertilise. Wrong! Whether you have sex standing, sitting, lying, upside down or in the sea you can still get pregnant. But you might not: I once heard of a contortionist who was so desperate to be a mum she used to stand on her head for ages after sex in the belief it might help her conceive. Sadly for her, it failed.

When a girl loses her virginity, there is blood everywhere and it hurts.

If it was that bad do you think we would all be so keen to be deflowered? Making love for the first time CAN be painful for a girl if she is not completely aroused (it can also be painful for non-virgins if their lovers are inexperienced or insensitive enough not to know when the moment is right). But not all of today's virgins need fear bloodshed due to the tearing of the hymen—the skin across the entrance to the vagina—because by the time they're ready to start their sex life, many have torn it thanks to strenuous sport or the use of tampons. The least painful way a girl can lose her virginity is to a caring and skilful lover who will know that it will be as painless as possible for her if she is aroused to fever pitch first.

If you masturbate you'll grow hair on your palms and you could go blind or mad or both.

Masturbating—that is, giving yourself pleasure by rubbing your genitals—is a normal, healthy pastime. It relieves sexual tension, helps you discover what your body enjoys—and most people have tried it before they are out of their teens. Many sexperts recommend it as a way of practising your love technique so you can let a partner know which touches turn you on. In less enlightened times, people used to try to stop children masturbating by telling them the one about the hairy palms or that they would wear out their sex organs. But now we know better.

You can't get pregnant if the penis does not enter the vagina.

Whoops. You would be quite unlucky but if only a few drops of your lover's semen spilled in your pubic area, anywhere near the entrance to the vagina, his sperm could make their way to your uterus and fertilise an egg. When you realise there are millions of sperm in every teaspoonful of semen; that it only takes ONE to make a baby and that once released sperm stay active for about two days, this type of accidental pregnancy doesn't seem so impossible.

Men are always ready for sex—they can have an erection any time.

A woman could be forgiven for thinking this if the lusty male in her life is clearly roused every time he looks at her. But even the most ever-ready males suffer power failure at some stage. It usually happens if he's been working too hard and has become tired and stressed or worried about his job. Or if he's been drinking too much and is suddenly hit by brewer's droop. Or if he's feeling guilty about having sex with someone he shouldn't. Whatever the cause, the answer is: don't panic. Worrying about it makes it worse. And once he's that depressed about lack of performance he'll find it harder and harder to get harder and harder.

Good sex means making yours and your partner's orgasms coincide.

It's wonderful if you can make it happen just the way it does in steamy novels, with the two of you going at it like a runaway train till the world explodes in a dazzle of stars and you fall back exhausted and satisfied. That's the way it is in fiction but in real life it is rather different. Some people never manage it, some achieve it occasionally, some make it happen most of the time and a tiny group reckon they crack it every time. But whatever you do in bed, if it leaves both of you with that warm, satisfied glow of total pleasure, it's Good Sex.

Orgasms are automatic for women if they know what they're doing in bed.

If only. Most young women need a good bit of sexual practice before discovering how to achieve orgasmic sex every time—or every time they want it. They very rarely enjoy this physical treat the first time they make love—which some find quite a letdown, considering all the hype surrounding the Big O.

Women only have orgasms if you stimulate their clitoris.

The clitoris seems to have become the push-button answer to perfect sex. Some women find they cannot reach peak excitement unless their clitoris is massaged by their partner or themselves during actual intercourse. Some even believe that a woman will never work up to an orgasm from just the thrusting of a penis in her vagina. In fact, the good news is you can have an orgasm while having your toes sucked, your nipples nuzzled or, in some cases, the palm of your hand licked. And plenty of women will tell you that a well-operated penis can certainly make the earth move for them—as long as there's been some exquisitely executed foreplay beforehand.

Condoms spoil sex for men.

Most men would prefer not to have their most prized possession swathed in rubber as, they say, it diminishes their pleasure during sex. However prostitutes, whose lives and livelihoods depend on keeping free of sexually transmitted diseases, especially AIDS, say they've learned to put condoms on unsuspecting male customers by using their mouths. And the men don't notice till afterwards. What men—and women—find most discouraging about condom use is having to interrupt the most exciting moments of sex play to put it on. So any way that can be done without a break in play will keep everyone happy. They say you can learn to put a condom on with your mouth by practising on a cucumber.

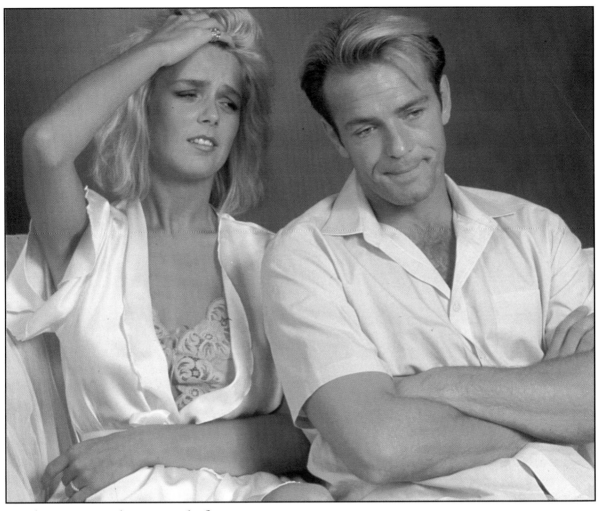

Myth: men are always ready for sex

Men don't need foreplay.

So many women have complained about the wham-bam-thank-you-ma'am style of loving, where foreplay consists of dropping your trousers, that men haven't been able to get a word in about their own needs for preliminaries. Yes, that man who looks as if he has a python trying to escape from his trousers would like some gentle, loving handling from you. He doesn't relish being grabbed by the goolies any more than you like having your boobs scrunched by a hairy hand before you've had time to say 'Had a nice day, dear?'

Women don't ejaculate.

It doesn't happen in the same way it does with men, but some women release a spurt of fluid when they climax. It is thought to come from a female version of the prostate gland just inside the vagina.

Men can't have multiple orgasms.

It has emerged that Mother Nature has, after all, been very fair about this. Californian researchers clocked one record-breaking male achieving a gasp-making 16 orgasms in an hour. They say this was not done with rests in between but in a series culminating in ejaculation. Phew!

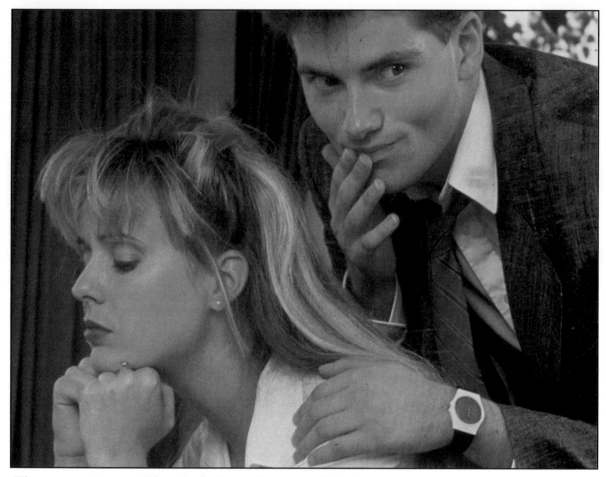

The woman in your life only feels randy some of the time.
At other times she'd rather read a book.

Women who have big vaginas have had a lot of lovers.

Some men really believe this but it's as silly as thinking men with giant penises have made them grow by using them a lot. Some people's equipment is just bigger than others. It should be remembered that the vagina is so elastic it can stretch to let a baby enter the world through it. And most babies are vastly bigger than penises.

Men with big hands/feet/noses also have big penises.

As anyone who's ever spent any time on a nude beach will vouch, the size of a man's other bits has absolutely nothing to do with the size of his wedding tackle. A man with size 12 feet can have a size-unimpressive penis and so can a man with an outsize hooter.

Whatever women say to the contrary, they really want sex all the time.

Anyone who believes this has been reading too many zipper-rippers about sexually voracious women who fulfil men's fantasies by panting for sex every waking moment. Sorry guys, the woman in your life only feels randy some of the time. At other times she'd rather read a book, watch a movie or paint her nails. And this is quite normal.

Size doesn't count.

Not quite true. In fact, size does matter when a penis is too big or too small. Then it can be a problem making love, specially if it's too long and pushes against a woman's cervix. If it's abnormally small (and this is very rare) it won't give a woman much of a thrill either. Average length is six and a half inches when erect but as the average vagina also stretches to about six and a half inches when it's ready for sex, average is all a man needs to be. But some women do like to *see* a whopping one and if length doesn't matter, circumference certainly does. A thick one is mostly more stimulating in action than a thin one.

You can't get pregnant if you aren't having periods.

Yes you can. A girl can get pregnant just before her first period and a woman can get pregnant before her periods have resumed after she has had a baby. Once ovulation has taken place—an egg has been released from an ovary and travelled to the womb, ready for possible fertilisation—you can get pregnant. This happens midway between two periods—or, in the case of the first period, about two weeks beforehand.

The amount of semen a man ejaculates at a time could fill a milk bottle or at least a cup.

This is a total exaggeration, wishful thinking or plain misinformation. It may seem like a fountain when it gushes out but is scarcely ever more than a teaspoonful.

Men cannot fake orgasms.

Plenty say they can and do. What they mean is, they may not ejaculate but they bump and thrust like crazy before shuddering to a groaning halt—and hope their partner may not notice the missing teaspoonful.

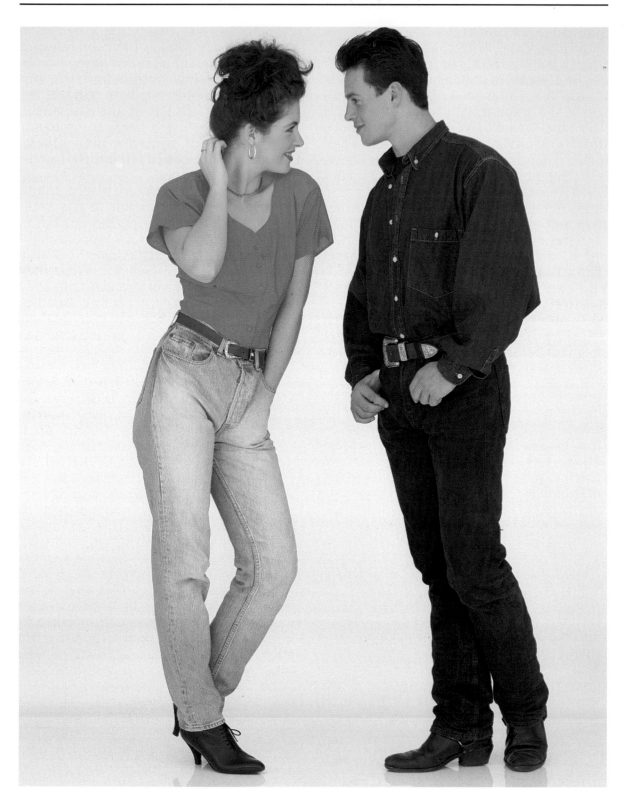

LOVE AND ATTRACTION
Magic—or can you turn it on?

Call it animal magnetism or just pure magic, it hits like a bolt from heaven and leaves your senses reeling. You look into someone's eyes, your pulses race and your legs feel useless.

It has nothing to do with whether you like them as a person—you can be sexually attracted to someone whom you know nothing or little about. And once you get to know that person, you may discover they don't appeal to you at all—you hate their views, their voice, their politics or the way they dress.

Sadly, sexual attraction isn't always mutual. You can be irresistibly drawn to someone who either doesn't know you exist or shows no sign of wanting to know you better. This is specially true of the kind of celebrities we'd all like to wrap ourselves around, sex icons like Mel Gibson, Sharon Stone, Kim Basinger, Tom Cruise. But it's also true of the girl or guy at the bus-stop each morning who never seems to be looking your way. And when they do, they look right through you.

Since forever, men and women have agonised over the mystery of why one person sets us quivering with desire and another leaves us as cold as a frozen cod fillet. The only thing you can say for certain is that you know when it happens and you know when it doesn't. Try to analyse what it is that excites you about someone and you are unlikely to be able to pinpoint any one quality. You may list a number of things like their green eyes, their dimples, their smile and the way they look out from under their long lashes. Or their sharp brain and the way they make you laugh. But then you might think of others who have these qualities yet don't appeal to you in the same way.

The most heart-tearing puzzle of all is why someone we fancy like crazy does not feel the same about us. We can't help thinking there must be something we can do to change the situation—dye our hair blonde, lose a stone, splash out on a new perfume or after-shave, learn to tap-dance or climb Everest. In Shakespeare's Midsummer Night's Dream, much of the plot revolves round the squeezing of a flower in the eyes of sleeping characters which causes them to fall madly in love with the first person they see on waking. Some people will try ANYTHING to attract the object of their desire.

Luckily for the future of the human race, we all fancy different aspects of potential lovers: one man will pant with lust at the sight of a big-breasted blonde while another will be far more excited by a slim, athletic brunette. To each his own, as they say. But there are certain features we all seem to agree on as desirable in others—which is why certain movie, music and sports stars have thousands steamed up at the sight of them.

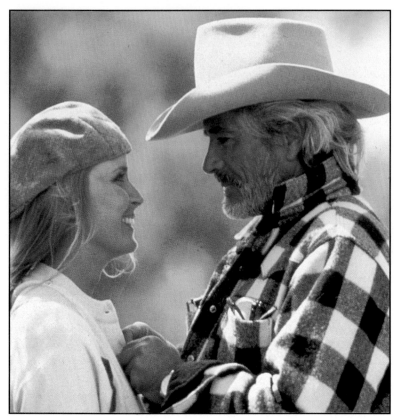

A trade-off often takes place—the age gap, say, will be compensated for by his maturity and wisdom. (John and Bo Derek)

Here are some ingredients of sexual attraction that scientists have been able to pinpoint:

BEAUTY

It may be in the eye of the beholder but if your face fits the generally accepted idea of what's currently thought attractive, you'll have instant appeal for many of the opposite sex. Experiments carried out in both Britain and America have found that good-looking men and women are nearly always favoured above those of average looks or those thought physically unattractive.

If your looks are above average, others will expect you to be above-averagely good-natured, intelligent, successful and happily married. You will be more likely to be a successful job applicant and others will trust you more, believing you are as good on the inside as you are on the outside.

It has also been found that most people marry partners whose level of looks is the same. That is, good-looking men and women marry each other; women with average looks marry men of average looks and plain Janes marry plain Johns.

But there are some blindingly obvious exceptions to this, where Beauty has ended up with the Beast. Very often, in those cases, a trade-off will have taken place—his ugliness, say, will be compensated for by enormous wealth or success. When a dazzlingly handsome man marries an unattractive woman, you will very often see that she is spectacularly rich, clever, aristocratic or has some other hugely desirable characteristic which makes up for her looks. Think of famous couples whose looks are a mismatch and the trade-off will almost certainly be obvious.

THE DIFFERENCE BETWEEN US

For a heterosexual, the most attractive feature of the opposite sex is, wait for it, they are different. Men are excited by the essentially female physical details and women are turned on by what men have got that they have not.

Because men were meant to hunt, fight and protect their women and children, their bodies are built specifically to do those jobs. So men have bigger hands and feet than women, more developed muscles, bigger shoulders and chests, bigger and

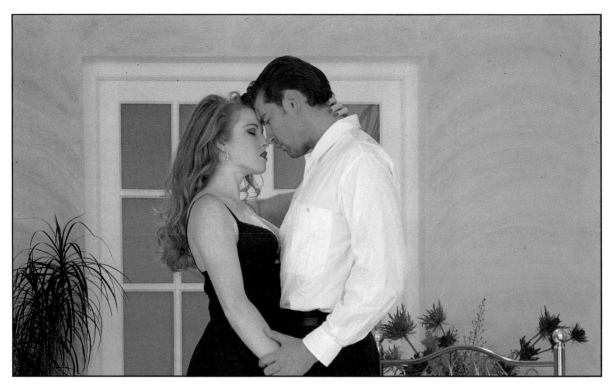

Women prefer men to be taller than them, though in a similar height bracket.

stronger jaws—and they are taller.

Women, designed for childbirth, have a wider pelvis, bigger buttocks, bigger breasts, more space between the tops of their thighs—and more fat.

Where the difference is pronounced—say, a man is taller, more big-jawed and broad-shouldered than average—he will have extra sex appeal. A woman with big breasts and curvy hips will have a lot of appeal for a lot of men.

But luckily for the rest of us, there are plenty of women panting with lust for men with slender, unmuscular bodies and pretty faces—and hordes of males turned on by girls with slim hips and no use for Wonderbras.

HEIGHT

In the sex stakes, being tall gives a man a head start over his shorter rivals. That's because extra height is prized in Western society, not only as an attribute of maleness but as a stamp of success. Research has found that taller men get better-paid jobs and more respect—if he is tall, people presume he is in authority.

Women prefer men to be taller than them, though in a similar height bracket. This means shorter than average women mostly pair off with short-ish men who are slightly taller than themselves. And very tall women tend to end up with even taller men.

When a very short man finds the even shorter woman of his dreams, it has been found they often marry very soon after—presumably because it's too good an opportunity to miss.

EYES

Women's eyes are mostly bigger and rounder than men's and where nature has been less than generous, a woman can make up the difference with cosmetics if she wants to add to her sex appeal. Tests have found that humans are instinctively drawn to a pair of circles with a dot in the middle, and the more the dots fill the circle, the more interested people become. This is thought to be why nature designed babies' eyes and pupils to be large in proportion to their heads—they need to

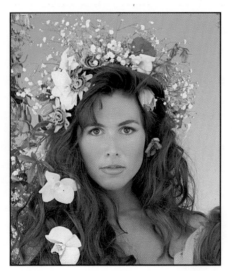 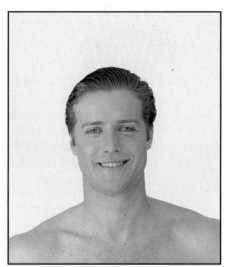

Women's eyes are mostly bigger and rounder than men's

look adorable to bring out our caring side, ensuring their welfare.

Women's eyes probably have the same vulnerability factor for the same reason— indeed, it's been found over and over that when a man looks into a woman's eyes and sees enormous pupils he is automatically drawn to her.

It has also been found that the pupils of people's eyes grow bigger when they see something that attracts or excites them.

In one famous test, a group of men was shown a pair of identical photographs of a girl, one of which had been altered by enlarging the pupils of her eyes. The men were more than twice as excited by the picture with the large pupils, according to observers who monitored the expansion of the men's pupils. Yet most were not aware of any difference between the photographs—so their reaction must have been pure instinct.

In Mediaeval times, women used the drug belladonna (Italian for beautiful woman) to increase the size of their pupils and make them more desirable.

The first contact we have with another person is when we look at them. And if they catch us looking interested and like the look of what they see— Bingo! it's the first sign of sexual attraction. Notice that their pupils have expanded and you know they fancy you.

SMELL

Mmmm, just a whiff of someone who crosses your path can be enough to fill you with longing to know them better. Smell is such a powerful part of sexual attraction that the whole perfume industry has been based on trying to bottle the elusive secret of what drives two people into each other's arms.

If only it was just a matter of splashing on that after-shave or squirting that ferociously expensive fragrance behind your ears and knees.

Women are particularly sensitive to the scent of a man, being brought almost to swooning point by an odour that attracts them (and, it has to be said, sent sprinting away from a pong that says he hasn't washed much lately). But the smell that has them sniffing with delight and desire is not usually something you can buy, but rather a natural sexual scent known as pheromones.

Animals have it secreted in special glands. When the female of the species gets a whiff of the male's pheromones, she gets excited and her own pheromones send out the signal that she's ready for sex. It is now thought humans operate in the same way via sex glands in the armpit and genital areas. However, we have done our best to suppress the system by dousing our bodies with deodorants, anti-perspirants, perfumes and the like, specifically aimed at killing natural body odours.

However, nature no doubt has its way occasionally which might explain why, for no reason you can explain, you suddenly feel sexy stirrings in the direction of someone you might otherwise not have noticed.

The other way we sometimes turn on to another person's special smell is when it evokes a memory of a person or event that was sexually arousing in the past. It might be the odour of a past romantic setting—the smell of wood and salt air from a boat, of jasmine and oranges from a Mediterranean courtyard—or someone's favourite perfume which lingered on clothes and in rooms long after they'd left. Our memory is said to be jolted far more strongly by smell than by sight or sound.

LIPS
You may think a lush pair of lips looks kissable merely because of their sensuous shape or inviting rosy colour.

The famous author and zoologist Desmond Morris says that a woman's lips echo the shape of her genitals which, like those of female monkeys, redden and swell when she's ready for sex. But, unlike monkeys who run round on all fours showing their readiness to their mates, women have to keep this obvious visual signal well hidden. Lipstick, he says, is not just a beauty aid but a sex signal.

And it has been proven by researchers that men think lipstick a sign of frivolity and sexiness. In an American experiment, male college students had to spend ten minutes talking to six females, only three of whom wore lipstick.

Afterwards they judged that the lipstick wearers were less interested in their work and more keen on the opposite sex than the bare-lipped girls. Yet in some cases they had seen the same girls, with and without lipstick. None of the men had noticed the presence or absence of lipstick.

DON'T GET THE WRONG IDEA
Instant impressions of another person are easy to form—but they can be so wrong. We all make judgements based on assumptions about all sorts of things, from hair colour ("blondes have more fun") and nationality ("Frenchmen are sexy") to similarity to ourselves ("you're like me..."). It is a kind of shorthand method we all use to work out quickly whether we want to get to know

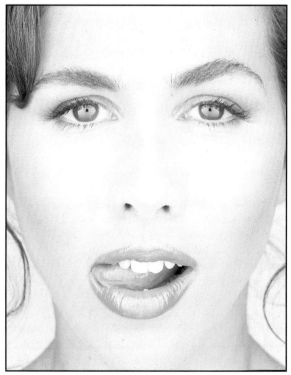

Lipstick is not just a beauty aid but a sex signal.

someone better. It gets called intuition, sixth sense and even love-at-first-sight— but basically it is rarely much more accurate than being blindfolded and trying to find your number in the phone book.

Psychologists have listed six main ways in which we tag people with characteristics they may or may not have.

1. Stereotyping: We all learn to categorise people the moment we're introduced, according to the information instantly available. If he's Italian, he's hot-blooded; if she's an air hostess she'll be an easy lay; if he's a Cockney he'll be street-wise; if she's showing acres of flesh she's ready, willing and available for sex.

2. Personality Pairs: Because someone has one generally admired characteristic, we automatically link it with another. If someone is physically strong, say, we presume they are brave. If someone is attractive though silent we often deduce that they are a deep thinker and highly intelligent. They may, in fact, turn out to be shallow and dumb.

3. Personal Superstitions. We've all got pet theories about people we fancy, based on the past. If you once had a fling with an artist obsessed by your toes, you'll expect all artists to be toe-fanci-

ers. If a bank clerk once cheated on you with your best friend, you'll never trust a bank worker again.

4. One-off Incidents: At the moment you first set eyes on someone they happen to be throwing a wobbly over the fact their car has been vandalised. Or perhaps they look pale and gaunt because they've stayed up late studying. Whatever the first impression, you keep that view of them as a true picture. So you label the first as hysterical and the second as frail and unhealthy forever more.

5. Buck-passing. If you've got a secret sexual fear you may cope with it by making

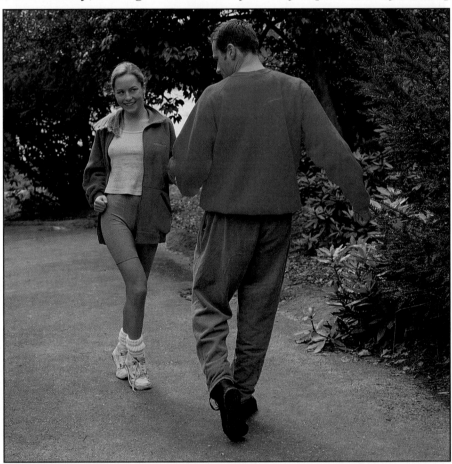

Instant impressions of another person are easy to form—we all try to work out quickly whether we want to get to know someone better.

yourself believe it's not you but the other person who is worried about being gay or is terrified of sex. This is a theory known as 'projection', which seems logical but is hard to prove.

6. You're like me. If you're addicted to Mars bars and you see someone else chomping on one, you take it for granted they are like you in every other way. Or if you meet someone who comes from the same small town as your dad, you expect to relate to them in the same way you got on with your dad. It's easy to get carried away and presume more things in common than there really are.

Sexual Attraction—Things People Say

"I really like fat, ugly men. They're always nicer than the good-looking ones."

"I first noticed his cheekbones because they were like they'd been hewn out of rock. After that I was fascinated by his silence. He was so quiet I couldn't help wondering all the time what he was thinking. I thought he must be really bright."

"I like blondes. That's always the first thing I notice about a woman. Then I notice her legs, then I probably look at her eyes."

"Hair is what I go for, every time. Flowing hair. But there are a lot of disappointments—like when they turn round and show their face. And then you hear their voice—oh dear!"

"I always go for the one in a group who is the most talented, the most funny, the most good-looking or witty. I think it's partly because I'm embarrassed to attach myself to people so I go for the one who's guaranteed acceptable. Or you could say I just go for skinny boys with curly hair."

"He was a musician and I think I was spellbound by his creative energy at first. But after about four months without a proper conversation, I realised he was actually quite boring."

"She had specks of paint on her face and hair and dark circles under her eyes. It really brought out my caring kind of soppy side."

"Her thighs were mind-blowing. Muscley. I couldn't take my eyes off them—it was all I could do to keep my hands off them."

"He had green eyes that turned up at the corners and he seemed a bit arrogant. He was clever and he knew it."

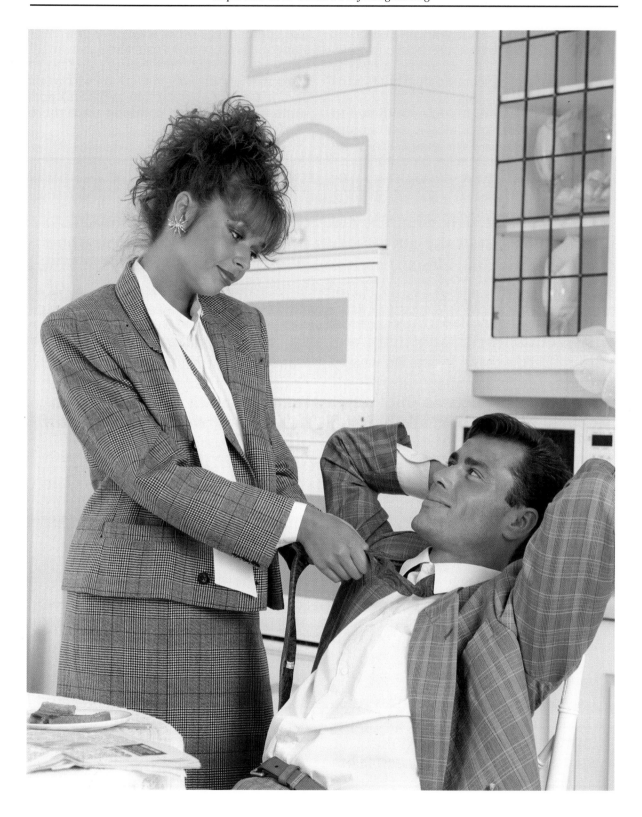

COME-ONS
Can it hurt to flirt?

Flirting is such good fun it should be taught in school. As a game, it's a much more useful skill than cricket or hockey (you don't need a whole team to play it, either—just two of you). And, unlike most other sports, you can keep at it till you're 100.

For some of us, it's never more than a sexy come-on to brighten the day but to others it verges on an art form, a technique to be polished and perfected. And then there are those who frown on flirting as a dangerous type of teasing. And those who would never think of being so frivolous—it's a meaningful relationship or nothing.

Yes, flirting is what you make it, any or all of the above. The best thing about it is that it's an easy way to start a relationship that may lead to something—or nothing.

Flirting can tell someone you like the look of them—and give them the opportunity to return the compliment. It is a way of finding out in a light-hearted way whether there is a spark between you and someone you fancy. And of opening up the possibility of taking things further.

Flirting also keeps a sparkle in a long-term relationship, where it tells your mate you still find them the sexiest animal in the universe. Or it can spice up the agenda of the working day by taking your mind off serious matters for a brief moment or two. And there's nothing like a saucy, harmless flirtation with a customer or salesperson to get anything from cabbages to used cars at the price you want.

The main thing about being a flirt is: to get the most out of it, you have to be good at it. Fine art or special skill, you need to understand the techniques and tactics.

So here goes with the Super-sexcessful Flirts' Foundation Course.

Lesson 1: The Idea.

The aim of the game is to have fun, make friends and maybe find romance. It is about getting yourself noticed and liked at the same time—by someone who attracts you. Anyone can do this, as long as they are confident and outgoing enough to make the first move. Think about it: you can flirt—outrageously or subtly, depending on your personality—or you can hang about waiting for others to make a move in your direction.

Okay, so you're shy. So too, probably, is that gorgeous stranger you are desperate to know better. So who's going to approach whom? Or are you just going to sit tight and hope for a mystery force to drive you towards each other? Or worse, watch a braver person move in and snatch Gorgeous from right under your nose? Of course you're not. So take a few deep breaths and get ready to go flirting.

All you need is a winning smile and a bit of wile 'n guile. You should also only flirt when

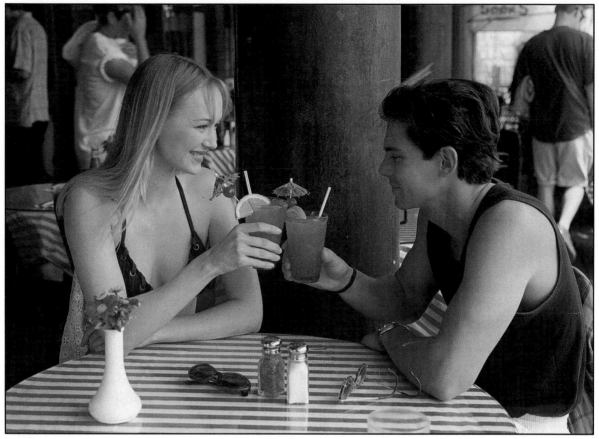

Catch someone's eye, then give a sunny smile that says you're warm and friendly

you're feeling good about yourself—when you know you're at your gold medal best and anyone would be a fool not to fancy you.

And don't take it too seriously. It's no major blow if someone doesn't swap smiles or phone numbers. Move on to someone who does. Remember, you're not walking the streets asking people to marry you, you're just being friendly.

Oh, and it's better not to get up the courage for your flirting debut by getting legless first. It's embarrassing to others at the time—and to you, when you sober up.

Lesson 2: The Moves.

You can do it with a word, a look, a gesture, anything that rouses someone's curiosity about you. And makes them want to know more.

Here are some basic moves—it's up to you to think of brilliant flirting strategies of your own.

• Catch someone's eye, then give a sunny smile that says you're warm and friendly—but not too friendly. If you hit them with your let's-go-to-bed look in the first seconds, you may frighten them to death. Or make them pounce on you.

• Compliments are always a winner, but don't overdo the flattery or they'll think you're taking the mickey. It's over the top to tell him his body could have been sculpted by Michelangelo if he's just lost a couple of inches round the waist. Praise his willpower instead.

• Hello is the first thing you say to someone so say it with enthusiasm, as if you're thrilled to meet them. If you sound bored or nervous they'll just want to move on.

• A witty T-shirt, funny tie, knockout hat or amazing piece of jewellery is a great conversation starter. Wear something odd and everyone HAS to ask you about it.

• Read newspapers and magazines that are full of off-the-wall items and quirky stories you can trot out when the talk gets dull. You'll get chalked up as an entertaining, interesting person.

• Be sure to catch the name of the person you hope to attract when you're introduced. Use it in conversation—they'll be flattered you're that interested.

• If you're female, fiddle with your hair, a necklace or ring (specially if you've been told you have pretty hands). Or let a shoe dangle from your toes. Signals like this are never missed by men.

• If you're male, carry a big book on your favourite subject—she won't be able to resist asking about it.

• If you get to shake hands with the object of your fascination, put in an extra squeeze of the fingers—just to show you're REALLY pleased to meet them

• After seeming easy-to-get, play hard to get. Once you've got them hooked, back off. They'll wonder what's going on and be even more intrigued.

• Blow a kiss then clap your hand to your mouth in mock-horror, as if you've just realised it wasn't the person you thought it was. Then you can go over to them and explain, so you can both share the funny side.

• Speak in a soft, husky voice as if you've got a touch of laryngitis. Whoever you're talking to will have to lean close to hear you.

• Look at the person you fancy while whispering in someone else's ear. Smile as you do it and it will seem you're saying something flattering about the one who matters.

• Ask for advice, opinions, views on life from someone who looks interesting to you. Not only will you find out enough to decide if you want to know them better, they will be pleased at the chance to talk about themselves.

• Once you've caught someone's eye, look away briefly then take a second look. They'll know you're interested and may make a move to know you better.

• Don't let it be known, the moment you've met someone new, that you're available. Keep them guessing. Mention something you did by saying "we" did whatever it

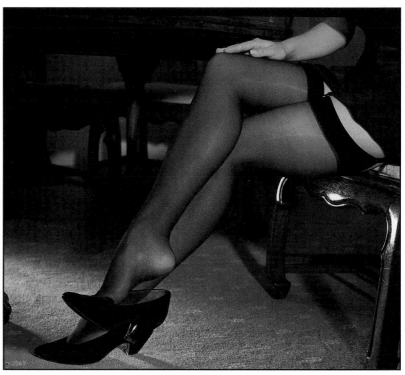

Let a shoe dangle from your toes. Signals like this are never missed by men.

was—you could be talking about your friend, flatmate, brother or sister but they will be desperate to discover how free you are.

• Mirror the moves of that beautiful person you're standing near at a party or in a crowded bar. Hold your glass in the same hand, place your feet in the same position, sip when they do. Do it subtly and not as if you're mimicking them as a joke. It'll take a while for them to become aware of you, but they certainly will. And they'll be appreciative, because everyone feels good about being copied.

• Make a small move towards the person you feel attracted to—either lean slightly nearer to hear what they're saying, take a tiny step or move closer on the sofa you're sharing. But be careful not to invade their space by getting too close for comfort. If they immediately back off to keep the dis-

tance between you, you've pushed your luck.

• Send a postcard to the one you fancy—at work if you don't know their home address. Make it a funny one. And don't forget to sign it.

Lesson 3: The Rules.

Subtlety is the key to flirting. You don't have to jump up and down and make a fuss to be noticed. Listening to someone intently, as if they are talking only to you, is one of the most flattering gestures you can make.

You don't need outrageous, clever or original chat-up lines. It's not what you say, it's how you say it. Asking the time or seeking directions is a good enough way to start talking to someone.

• Only flirt with one person at a time—you don't want the whole room elbowing each

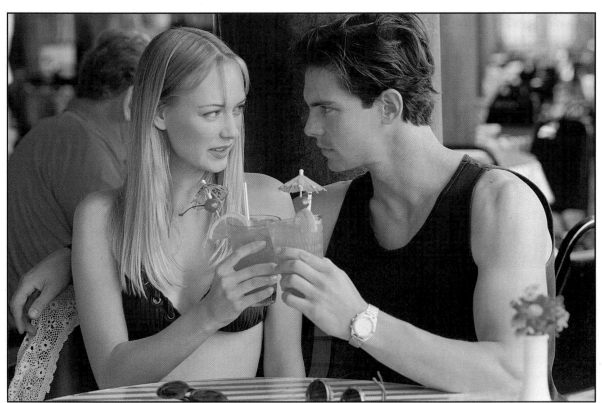

Make a small move towards the person you feel attracted to—lean slightly nearer to hear what they're saying.

other to reach your side.

• Always try to look as if you're having a good time, even if you're not. People are attracted to those who are clearly enjoying life—and turned off by those who look glum, grumpy or sorry for themselves.

• Don't let your eyes wander restlessly round the room when someone is talking to you. They will immediately register that you're not interested in them.

• Don't flirt if you don't mean it. It's no good giving someone the strong message that you'd drop everything and everyone for them, then acting surprised or offended when they try to take you up on it.

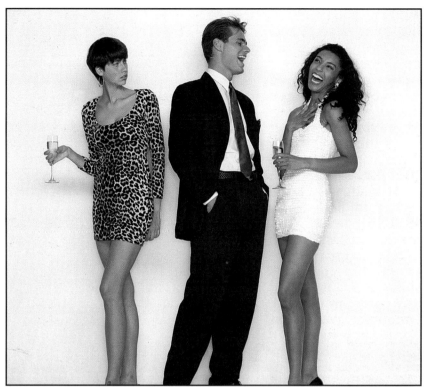

Don't envy that person you know who is a brilliant flirt and always surrounded by admirers—copy them.

• When you're complimented on your dress, your smile or your taste in ties, don't say, "Oh you've got to be joking" and dismiss the well-meant words. Say "Thanks. I appreciate it, coming from someone with your immaculate style."

• Wear your best clothes as much as possible instead of leaving them in the wardrobe for special outings. Why not look the best you can every day?

• Don't envy that person you know who is a brilliant flirt and always surrounded by admirers—copy them. Watch what they do, what they say, how they move and work out what it is that's so appealing. If you don't know anyone in real life who's flirty and fun, find someone on telly or in a favourite movie whom you'd like to be like.

• Don't hide away in corners or in places where you think you'll be unobtrusive. You have to be noticeable if you're hoping for a flirting match.

• Flirting is harmless. If you think things are going in a direction you don't like, it is in your power to stop the flirtation and move away

• Always flirt when there are more than just the two of you around, in case your action gets taken the wrong way

• Try to avoid flirting with anyone who has had too much to drink—they'll almost certainly get the wrong message, since their brain will be fuddled.

• Flirting with the locals on foreign territory is dead dodgy. What you think is meaningless they may find threatening or offensive, depending on their culture. And if there's a language problem, that's likely to make things worse. An accepted gesture in one country is often an insult in another.

• Don't try to be shocking—you never know how easily people can be offended.

• Certain people should be avoided by flirts: door-to-door salespersons (you'll never get rid of them); police officers (unwise to take their minds off the job. And if that's what you're trying to do, you're wasting your time— they'll see right through it); priests (unfair temptation); other people's spouses and lovers (unless you want to make enemies); your boss (too obvious, too tacky).

Lesson 4: The Venues.

Where do you find dishy women and hunky men with whom to flirt away a few happy moments? Almost everywhere. You don't have to go anywhere special. Wherever you are, look around and seize every

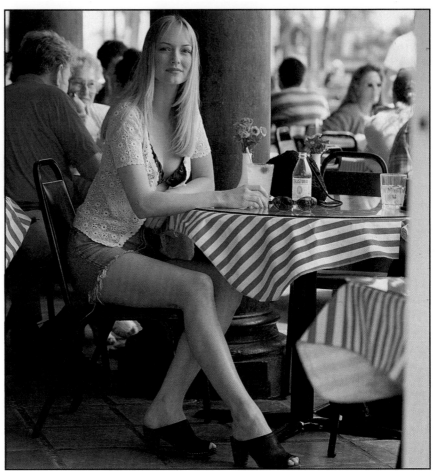

Wherever you are, look around and seize every chance to chat, smile or otherwise communicate

chance to chat, smile or otherwise communicate with a possible mate. For example:

Supermarkets—Ask her what you do with beansprouts; ask him to reach that can off the top shelf; ask her what sort of pooch she's bought the dogfood for; ask him if he's ever tried the Chicken Kiev.

Lunch and sandwich bars—Here's where you'll meet fellow workers in your area, snatching a bite. Ask her where there's a dry-cleaner nearby; ask him how he stays lean on bacon butties.

Cafés and restaurants—Ask about that headline in the newspaper she's reading; ask him what that exotic dish was that he just scoffed.

Queues—Brighten the most boring activity of all by chatting to someone nice beside you. Ask her if the Number 9 goes all the way to the city; ask him where he got that fabulous haircut; ask her what the papers said about the movie you're waiting to see; ask him what he thinks your chances are of getting a seat.

DIY shops—Handymen and women love to be asked for their help and advice. So why not make their day?

Sports stores—Notice whether they're trying on the cross-training shoes or the golfing spikes, then it's easy to strike up a conversation about the current state of the

British Open or when the next charity marathon takes place.

Travel agents—Tell her you're thinking of the Caribbean and ask if she's been there; ask him if the windsurfing is good in Turkey or if he's tried back-packing in Hungary.

At traffic lights—Great place to check out Gorgeous in the VW Golf. Wink, wave, blow a kiss, hold up a card with your phone number on it.

Newsagents—Spot the special interest magazines he's browsing then sidle up and ask what you should buy for your brother who's a wannabe pilot. Or ask her what's the best mag to help you decorate your bedroom.

Garages—Everyone cares about their cars: he wants to impress with his, she just wants hers to keep going without a hassle. Ask him how many mpg he gets; ask her what her Other Car is.

Flirting with the one you love

Just because that someone special is yours-all-yours it doesn't mean they don't want their ego tickled with a little flirting.

•Keep them boosted with daily doses of compliments and loving messages.

•Plant a kiss on a card and pop it into his wallet or her handbag.

•Gently pinch their bottom in public when no one's looking.

•Swap secret smiles when you're out in public, to let everyone know you belong to each other.

•Write "I love you" in make-up on the bathroom mirror or in dust on their car windscreen.

•Tell them the naughty thoughts you were having when you were waiting to meet them.

•Phone and tell them you'd like to try a certain sex fantasy when you get home.

•Write an outrageous message and slip it into their pocket so they'll find it when they're away from you.

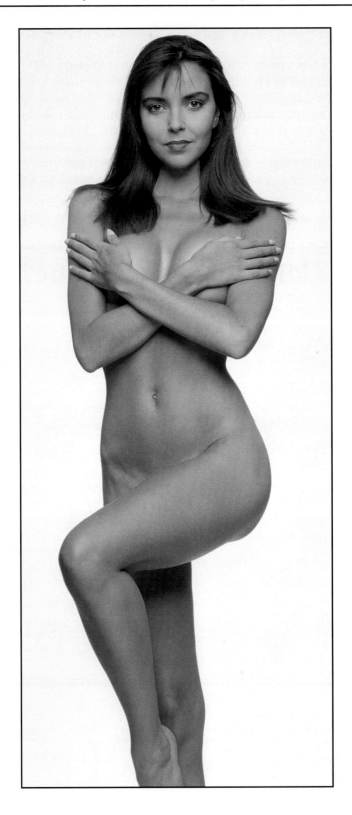

BODYTALK

How we move from date to mate

When you meet someone you like, it seems easy and natural to move from the getting-to-know-you chat to a friendly touch on the arm, from holding hands to kissing, from snogging to full sex. With some people it happens the first time they meet; with others it takes weeks or months. It is a complex ritual and one which separates us from other animal life—most other beasts don't mess about so much when choosing a lover.

There are ten basic steps from the moment you see someone you fancy to when you fall in love. And most couples need to go through all the steps before becoming lovers, according to the zoologist Desmond Morris, who identified man's ten-point mating routine in his book *Intimate Behaviour*.

So even those who claim love at first sight will be whizzing through the ritual on Fast Forward, from that first heady moment when they spot each other across a crowded bar to when they slip between the sheets to consummate their meeting.

Each step increases a couple's intimacy level by a notable degree—when you go from just liking the look of each other to asking 'Haven't we met somewhere before?' that's progress. And at each move forward there is a chance for one or both to decide enough's enough, that's as far as it goes.

That is how nature balances physical attraction and emotional closeness, so we don't end up jumping into bed with people who make us feel queasy over our cornflakes next day. (Next year, maybe—but that's another issue.)

It's a bit like playing snakes and ladders. You inch your way forward, hoping not to be rebuffed and sent sliding back down a snake to square one. If you only land on ladders, you'll be okay: you can go from seeing someone you fancy to scoring, without a hitch.

There are two vital rules if you want to win the mating game:

There's no hurry. You can take either months or minutes to play from start to finish.

Don't try to skip any steps—most people need to take them one at a time on their way to becoming lovers.

Ready to play? Look around to find a possible partner...

Step One—Wow! Seeing is fancying. The most fleeting sight of someone can send you into a spin when your brain registers that you like what you see. The minute your eye takes in that virile male or full-blown female figure with its sexy walk, colouring that could have been created by Renoir and a smile straight from heaven, your brain tells you there's someone just made for you.

If you take a second, closer look, you may

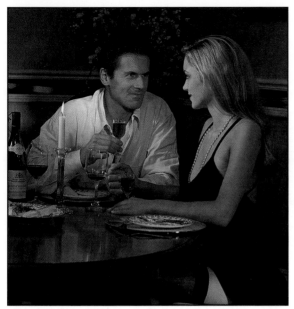

Gazing into someone's eyes is a strong sign of interest which tells them you like what you see.

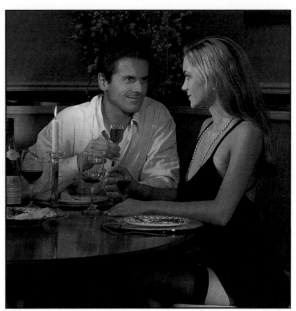

Your partner won't be listening to what you say so much as warming to the sweet tone of your voice.

decide that it's not Mr or Mrs Wonderful after all. In which case the game stops here—and you're on the lookout again.

What you may not have realised is the reason you noticed this god or goddess: it was not an accident they caught your eye, it was deliberate. When we see someone we fancy or imagine is attracted to us, we instinctively preen to show off our best points. We thrust out our chests, smooth our hair, lick our lips, walk with a wiggle. It all says: 'Hey, look at me, I'm desirable, available and within reach.'

Step Two—The eyes have it. If you can't take your eyes off the gorgeous being you've just discovered, sooner or later they'll catch you looking. That's when you'll feel a blush of embarrassment and the strong desire to dive under the nearest table. You will probably both turn quickly away at this point.

The next time your eyes meet you may look a fraction longer at each other, smile in recognition and raise your eyebrows slightly. You may make a small move in each other's direction.

Gazing into someone's eyes is a strong sign of interest which tells them you like what you see. It is also an invitation to get to know you better. Men tend to look for longer at a woman who interests them than women do at a man they fancy. If someone's eyes are wide open, they like the look of you. If they look at you through half-open eyes, they are considering their options.

You know they're looking interested? This is the cue to move on to the next stage

Step Three—It's not what you say, it's the way that you say it. Here is where we all run through our stock of chat-up lines for something better to say than: "Do you come here often?" But you needn't worry too much. What the other person is hearing is whether you sound confident (you're talking loudly), a bit scatty (you're

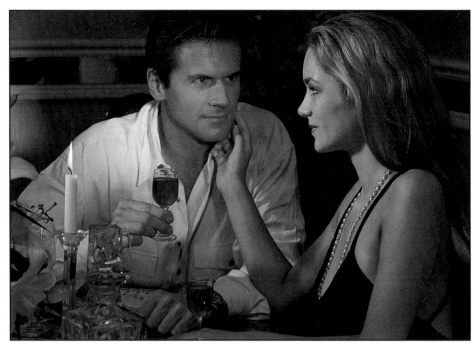

The first time you touch you may tingle from your finger-tips down to your toes.

danger of slipping, it was just that it was an excuse to make contact. It's a safe way of touching each other without being offensive or risking rejection. If someone doesn't want to be touched by you, they will somehow manage to avoid these harmless gestures.

Without having to put it into words, they'll be telling you: "I don't want to get any closer."

But if they greet your touch in a relaxed, easy way as if it was the most natural thing in the world, be reassured. They are happy to be moving closer to you. So you both know this could be the start of something special.

breathless), sexy (those deep, husky tones), weak (you're squeaking).

Dr Morris calls it grooming talk—monkeys groom each other as a gesture of friendliness, humans do it with words.

Your partner won't be listening to what you say so much as warming to the sweet tone of your voice and being melted by your smile.

Step Four—Tender touch. The first time you touch you may tingle from your fingertips down to your toes—but it won't be because there was anything intimate about this gesture.

You will have only shaken hands or timidly tapped an elbow, the sort of thing that goes on between acquaintances every day. Perhaps you took her arm to guide her over a pedestrian crossing, perhaps she reached out for support as she climbed down a steep path.

It wasn't that she needed help or was in

Step Five—Side Lines. You can tell things are hotting up when you feel relaxed about the side of your body touching the side of someone else's as you sit on a sofa, stand together or walk down the street.

If he puts his arm round your shoulder or links arms or holds hands it's a sign he's keen to get closer—but doesn't want to push his luck. Touching sides is friendly without being fresh. It is the beginning of physical togetherness and a sign you're becoming more than just good friends. You can judge the intimacy of this level of touching by realising you would not normally share this level of body contact with a same-sex friend.

Step Six—Time to Waist. Once your hands are on each other's waists, you're

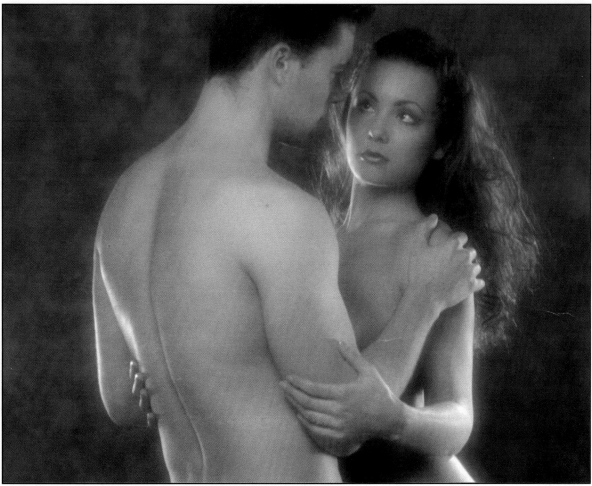

Your body gives off signals when you are ready for love

BODY SIGNS

Your body can be a giveaway when you'd rather it didn't tell tales. But there is nothing you can do about some signals your body gives out when you're longing for sex:

• Eyes glaze over and look dreamily into distance as the rest of the body tingles

• Skin pinkens as the temperature rises slightly

• Breath becomes shallower and faster as sexual excitement rises, followed by opening of the mouth to gasp in more air

• Skin prickles with sweat as it becomes warmer

• Heart starts to pound faster

• Extra sparkle in the eyes, which moisten with desire when the body is aroused

• Body smell intensifies as body warmth increases—so perfume, cologne, body lotion or after-shave scents will become more noticeable, as will natural body odours.

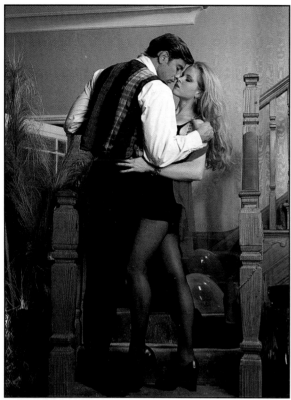

Once you're on kissing terms, your bodies will also be pressed together, front-to-front.

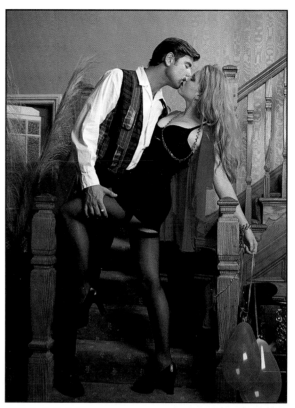

All inhibitions are gone as his hands seek out every secret part of her.

well on the way to being more than just good friends.

This is the first really sexy touch—judged by the fact that no man would ever put his arm round another bloke's waist, even if it was his best mate.

The hands are now creeping in the direction of more exciting contact with each other's bodies. This is the moment you have to decide whether you are ready for it, since now is the time to retreat if you are not.

Step Seven—Watch My Lips. Once you're on kissing terms, your lips pressed on each other's, your bodies will also be pressed together, front-to-front.

The longer you spend with your mouths locked together in kissing contact, the more likely your bodies will start to get sexy urges all over.

Human lips are a permanent sexy signal because, unlike animals' lips, they are curled back to show the puffy pink of their insides. Women's pouty lips, in particular, are said to be a replica of the sexy bits they don't expose to public view.

What both areas have in common, also, is super-sensitivity, growing red and swollen at moments of excitement—which is why mouth-to-mouth exercise is so electrifying.

But can you tell when to pucker up and go for that first super-charged smooch? You can get a fair idea by doing a bit of lip-reading. If their lips are shiny with moisture and you notice them being licked, go for it. And if they run the tip of their tongue very slowly and deliberately round the inside edge of their mouth, they are giving you an unmistakeable invitation to plant your lips on theirs.

Step Eight—Get Ahead. He strokes her

cheek, runs his fingers through her hair, fondles her neck. She caresses his neck and ears, trails a fingertip across his forehead.

Fondling someone's face with your hands is a very intimate gesture—couples do it as a first move towards passionate lovemaking. And honeymooners do it four times as often as long-wed couples.

The head and hair are immensely erotic, being prime erogenous zones in both men and women. So there are men who get shivers down their spine if a woman runs her fingers lovingly through their hair and women who go weak with desire when a man licks and nuzzles their ear-lobes or the base of their neck.

Step Nine—No Holds Barred. All inhibitions are gone as his hands seek out every secret part of her—and she does the same for him.

This is serious foreplay now: you both use your lips and tongues to explore each other's bodies in a frenzy of pleasure. It is the point of no return when you have both decided it is what you want.

You couldn't stop now, even if you wanted to.

Step Ten—You've mate it! Your bodies are locked together as passion builds and you are rocking and thrusting as one. This is the height of ecstasy when you reach a climax before sinking back in a state of happy exhaustion. Hopefully the earth has moved for both of you. The game is complete.

Your bodies are locked together as passion builds.

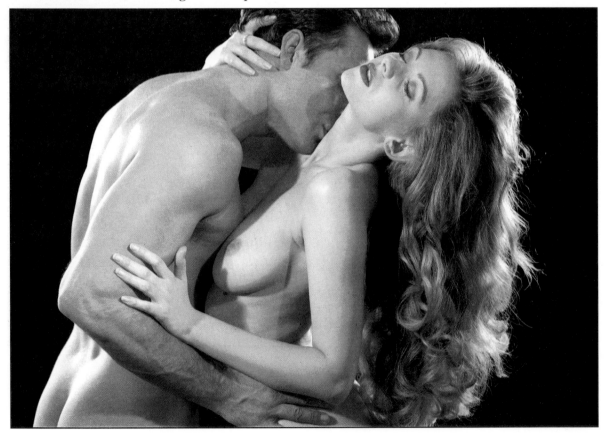

BODYSPEAK

The way you stand, sit and move tells all about the way you're feeling and what you're thinking, whether you want to be involved with the person by your side or whether you wish they'd go away. So if you want to know how another person feels about you, learn to read their body language. It will tell you more than words ever will.

Here is some basic body talk—and what it means:

• Arms crossed in front: If you are talking to someone who has their arms folded, it's likely they are not interested in you and are trying to block out what you say. It is also possible that they may be extremely shy and unable to communicate. Either way, it will be hard work getting through to them. If it's simply shyness that's the problem, you may notice them start to relax and open up, unfolding their arms as they warm to you.

• Legs crossed: If the leg on top is the one furthest from you, so its foot is pointed towards you, this person likes you and is happy to be with you.

• Hands on hips, chest thrust forward: They like you and want to get closer.

• Sitting, legs slightly apart: They fancy you and are ready to get physical

• Licking lips, tongue darting in and out: As far as they're concerned, you look lip-smacking good.

• Crossing and uncrossing legs (female): She wants you to find her sexy.

• Legs twined round each other: They are trying to lock their sexiest parts away from you—a sign of timidity and possibly disinterest.

• Shoulders tightly hunched: Doesn't want to know you and may be waiting for the first opportunity to vanish.

• Rubbing nose with finger: Whoever does this while talking to you is not telling the truth or trying to hide it in some way. Take what they say with a pinch of salt.

• Hand over part of the face: This person is trying to create a barrier between you

• Smoothing their hair: They like the look of you and hope you feel the same about them

• Gazing in your eyes: It's the look of love. Or lust. Or both.

• Low husky voice: Unless they're suffering from laryngitis, it's a sure sign they're having sexy thoughts about you

• Touching your arm, hand or knee: Trying to let you know they want to take things much further. If you shrink away, this will tell them you're not interested

• Smoothing skirt over hips (female): She's highlighting her curves to show off her desirability as a woman. She wants you to fancy her

• Standing with thumbs hooked in belt, feet apart (male): Fairly blatant way of saying he's ready for sex whenever you are.

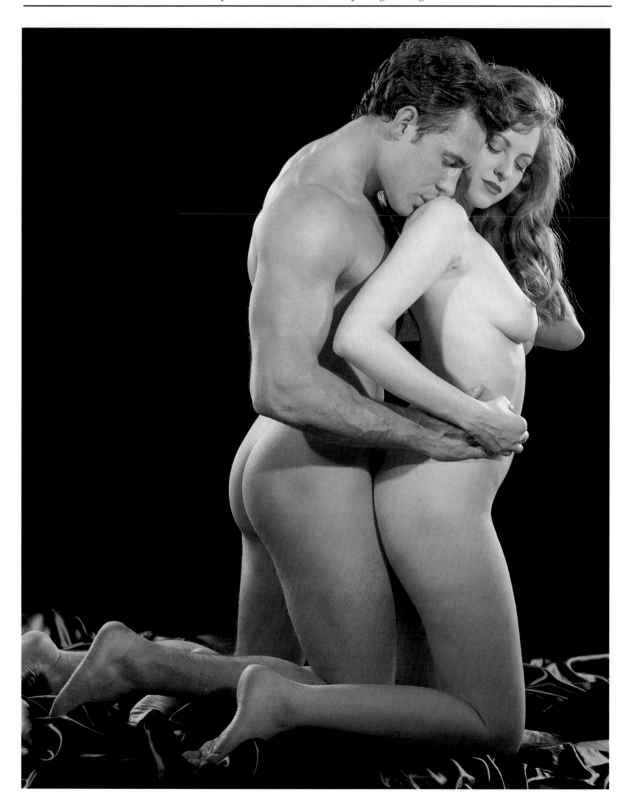

THE GEOGRAPHY OF LOVE
Chart your way to ecstasy

Bodies are a bit of a mystery to most of us, coming as they do in all shapes and sizes, colours and textures. And working as they do in similar yet strikingly different ways.

The one thing 99.9 per cent of people know about sex (I hope I'm not exaggerating) is that it's supposed to be wildly exciting when the man's sex organ, the penis, enters the woman's sex organ, the vagina. Most of us know this from an early age, having heard the rough (very rough) details in the school playground. We heard and told jokes implicitly describing this activity before we had any clear idea of what we were talking about (well it isn't cool to admit ignorance when you're four, is it?)

But even if you spent endless hours behind those bike sheds with a willing partner, minutely examining each other's bodily bits and pieces, you still ended up at 16, 18 or 27-and-a-half with only a shaky idea of the technique of making love. Like knowing the rules of tennis or football and owning the best kit for the game—but never having played much.

For instance, you may be able to name a person's parts from top to toe, draw a brilliant diagram of a cross-section of the male or female reproductive system—but faced with a beautiful naked specimen waiting to be played with, you find you're all thumbs, blushes and quivering apprehension.

What the text books so often don't tell you, among the drawings of internal organs, is how to handle the external organs, specially the stretches of skin not specifically labelled sexy bits. Basically, when you're studying a lover's body, there is the plumbing, with all its Latin names, and there are the pleasure zones. You need to understand the structure of the first before you can work your way sensitively round the second.

So let's take a short tour round Him and Her, to make sure you know your vagina from your vulva, your semen from your scrotum. It is absolutely vital to know exactly what is where, since your first experiences of a lover's body are usually in the dark and you are feeling rather than seeing your way. A bit like playing ping-pong in a blackout.

HER
Plenty of women are unfamiliar with the structure of their sexual equipment due to the difficulty of seeing it at close quarters. Tucked away as it is between the legs, hidden by a fuzz of pubic hair, it is best viewed sitting in front of a mirror with the legs parted. Not a pretty position to be caught in, so make sure the door's shut if you're the shy type.

Pubic hair is the first thing you see: can be sparse and downy but is mostly bushy and wiry-textured, like the contents of a

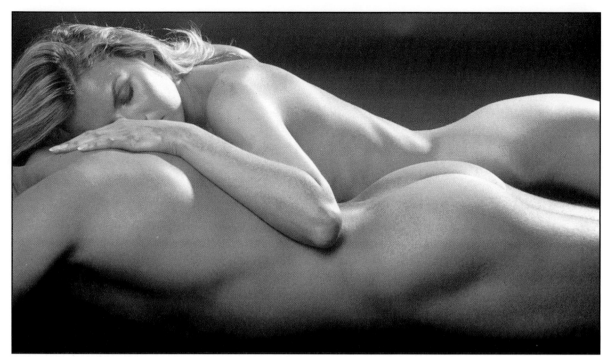

What the text books so often don't tell you, is how to handle the stretches of skin not specifically labelled sexy bits.

horse-hair mattress. It covers the vulva—the visible part of a woman's sex organs—and can spread in the direction of the navel as well as to the top of the inner thighs. Many women prefer it to be in a neat triangle so it doesn't hang out of their swimsuits in summer. Waxing, shaving or using depilatory cream to de-hair the 'bikini line' is the answer. Some couples find it very sexy for him to shave her pubic hair, either to tidy it or remove it entirely. But beware—it grows back as prickly as Velcro.

Vulva is the Latin word for the outer view of the female genitals. Not a word you may ever need to utter but there it is. It's what doctors say instead of 'naughty bits' and covers the whole area you can see.

Labia is Latin for lips and there are two pairs that guard the entrance to the vagina: the outer ones (labia majora) are fleshy and pale, with pubic hair on the outside and the inner ones (labia minora) are thin and red, without hair and rather loosely shaped.

The **clitoris** is the little button that holds the secret of sexual pleasure for a vast majority of women. It can be hard to find to the point where some women can't put their finger on their own. But a man who can't find his partner's clitoris is likely to leave her very frustrated. SO—it is at the top end of the inner lips, hidden by the folds where they meet and is only about the size of a small pea. But it does grow larger and harder and therefore easier to find when its owner is aroused. The clitoris is made of the same tissue as the penis and reacts in much the same way, that is, it grows erect when excited.

The **urethra** is the small opening through which urine leaves the body and it is not unknown for inexperienced lovers to mistake it for the vagina. Then they wonder why no babies are on the way. Some people look for thrills by poking things into this opening but it's definitely not recommended and could do serious damage.

The **vagina** is the opening between the urethra and the anus and is far more stretchy than the others, being able to extend from about three inches in length to nearly seven inches when its owner is sexually excited. It also stretches wide enough to let a baby out into the world so there is virtually no penis too big for a woman to welcome. But vaginas do feel pain when their delicate walls are rubbed too strongly, too energetically or too long by an unthinking lover. If a woman says intercourse is hurting and a man feels his penis not sliding easily in the vagina, it can mean that the juices that make the vaginal walls slippery for sex are not flowing—which means a woman may not be steamed up enough at this stage. More foreplay, please.

Breasts come in all shapes and sizes but no matter what their dimensions they are a strong source of sexual excitement, being full of nerve endings that the right caresses can coax to ecstasy. The breast itself is mostly fatty tissue surrounding a network of milk ducts which run into the nipple—and it's the nipple and surrounding pinkish skin that is the sexy bit. Lick and nibble this and she'll be in heaven—though, beware, there are times when the nipples are so tender they are out of bounds.

HIM

The **penis** is his most prized possession and the centre of all his sexual pleasure. What he mostly worries about is its size—which is mostly unimportant to a woman. It hangs limply when not excited but when stirred into life by sexual arousal it stretches and stiffens to its full size—about six and a half inches, on average. It also goes a darker, purplish colour due to the blood that rushes into it at this time. Its skin is fine and soft and if a woman strokes, holds, licks or handles it lovingly, its owner can hardly hold back from orgasm. The hole at the end of the penis is the entrance to the urethra through which urine is ejected and semen is ejaculated. Both fluids leave the body by the same route through the penis, though never at the same time. During sex, the bladder shuts off so there's no chance of urine mixing with semen.

The **testicles** are the two balls which produce both sperm and sex hormones and which hang in a sac, known as the **scrotum**, beneath the penis. This is a cunning device to keep the sperm at the right temperature, which is lower than the rest of the body's. When it's cold, the scrotum scrunches up so the testicles hang closer to

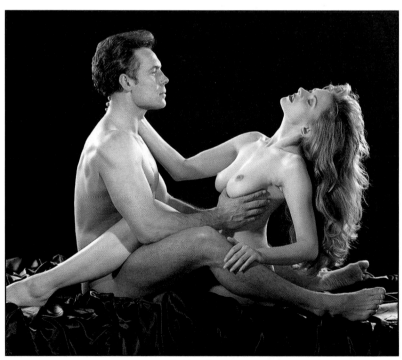

Breasts are full of nerve endings that the right caresses can coax to ecstasy.

the body and are kept warm. In hot weather, the scrotum sags so they hang lower and further from the body's heat. For some reason, the left testicle usually dangles lower than the right.

Semen is the fluid which a man ejaculates from his penis at the moment of orgasm. It is full of sperm, produced by the million in his testicles.

Foreskin is a loose fold of skin that covers the tip of the penis from birth, though some males have it cut away shortly after, in an operation known as circumcision. Religion or hygiene are mostly the reasons.

Whether the bulbous tip of his penis—the glans—is hooded by foreskin or exposed makes absolutely no difference to his sexual performance or pleasure.

THE PLEASURE ZONES

Apart from the obvious sex organs, everyone has other little nooks and crannies that thrill to the touch and throb with desire when given special attention by a sensitive lover. For some, having their ear-lobes nibbled is a five-star treat while for others, total ecstasy is reached when their fingers or toes are sucked.

The parts of the body that respond in this way are called the erogenous zones and every lover rates them differently. Men and women can share some of these pleasure points but different women will shiver with delight at different touches, one man's pleasure zone will be another's numb spot.

You have to feel your way lovingly round each new partner, watching how they spark up or switch off at your touch.

The following guided tour points the way to the commonest pleasure zones—and how to make them tingle.

HIS

Most men love to be pampered all over but it takes gourmet taste to know exactly which

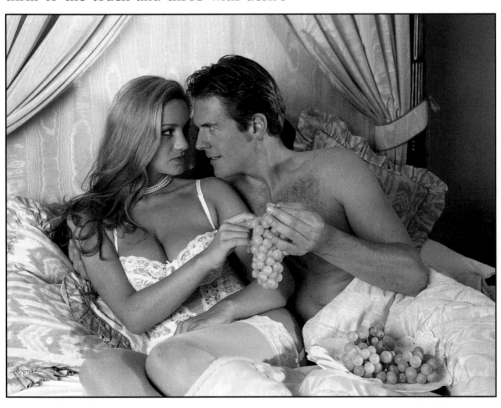

Everyone has little nooks and crannies that thrill to the touch and throb with desire when given special attention by a sensitive lover.

bits of his body to nibble and nuzzle, stroke and squeeze so he feels like your dish of the day and not a fast-food snack.

Head and hair
Treat his temples to a starter of nuzzles. Let your hot breath tickle his hairline as you run your fingers sinuously through his hair, gently massaging his scalp. Stroke his hair as you plant butterfly kisses over his brow with your own fluttering eyelashes. Then kiss the tip of his nose.

Ears
Savour the flavour of his skin as you run the tip of your tongue round the contours of his ear. Ever so gently bite his ear-lobe before blowing softly into his ear. While one ear is being treated by your lips and tongue, use your fingertips to trace the outline of the other one, tickling and caressing.

Neck
Love-bites don't have to leave vampire's marks all over him. Start just under his ear and work your way down his neck with little sucking kisses and nibbles. Stroke the other side of his neck with the spine-tingling tickle of your nails. Softly suck the back of his neck.

Lips
Feed off them as if they were your very last meal. Start with fast little kisses right round his lips, let your tongue dart teasingly in and out. Finally let your tongue tangle with his.

Chest and nipples
With stretched fingers, ease your hands over his chest feeling every muscle quiver under your touch. Notice how he expands with pleasure. Squeeze his breasts and tease his nipples with your fingernails, stroking the tips with feather touches till they start to harden. Then suck his nipples till they stand erect. Rest your head for a moment on his chest and listen to his heart race.

Back
Explore every muscle of his back with smoothing, probing fingers, helping to release the tensions of his day. Run your nails lightly down his spine to have him tingling with pleasure. Then kiss the back of his neck and run your tongue slowly down his back, vertebra by vertebra. Finish with a lingering kiss at the base of his spine.

Stomach
Plant soft kisses across his tum and dangerously near his dangly bits. Surprise him by blowing a raspberry in his belly-button. Then probe it slowly and thoroughly with your tongue.

Bottom
You don't have to be dainty in the way you relish his rear. Rub, stroke, pound and pummel it with both hands. Squeeze till it hurts, then let go. Give it gentle kisses and caresses, stroke it and admire the way his muscles tense. You could even bite his buttocks.

Thighs
Trail your nails down the inside of his thighs then nibble and lick your way back up again. Gently squeeze the back of his thighs, starting at the top and working down to the knees. Massage his front-of-thigh muscles then gently stroke his inside thigh.

Toes
Lick his toes like a row of lollipops then pop them in your mouth, one by one, and suck them till he shivers with joy. Massage under his arches at the same time and he will be in seventh heaven. But check first that he isn't ticklish, or you could get a nasty kick in the teeth.

HERS
Think of her body as a perfect instrument just made for you to play—and the better you know how handle it, the more beautiful music you will make. It is complex and takes practise to find the key parts.

Ears
Very sensitive, private parts which only those on the most intimate terms would dream of touching. They are delicate con-

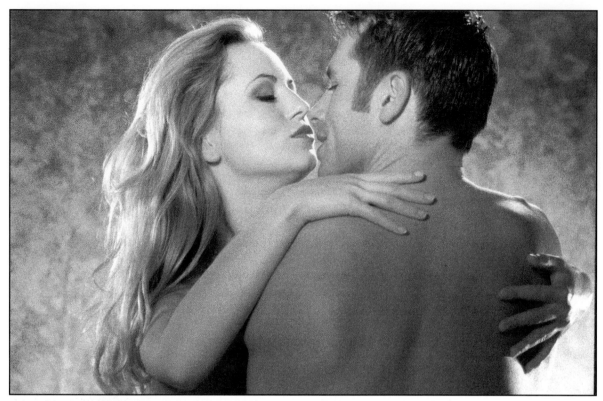

It's worth spending time trying every kind of kiss.

structions designed to pick up sounds and protect the fragile hearing mechanism. Trace the outline of her ear with the tip of your tongue, suck her ear-lobes and lick lovingly behind her ears to send shivers of delight through her whole body.

Neck

You'll set her spine tingling if you nuzzle your way lovingly round the back of her neck and kiss her lingeringly right in the nape. Then let your kisses flutter down her neck and round to her collarbone. The skin on the back of the neck is alive with nerve ends connected directly to the sex organs.

Lips and mouth

A totally erotic area, sizzling with nerve endings and imitating in shape a woman's more hidden sex organs. It's worth spending time trying every kind of kiss, from gentle lips-on-lips to the full tongue-tangler. While kissing her lips, dart your tongue quickly in and out of her mouth then run it right to the edges of her lips before letting it explore the whole inside of her mouth.

Navel

Ticklish, sensitive and often a very sexy place—but be gentle with it. Stroke the skin around it, lick it and blow gently round it. And for a real taste sensation, fill it with honey or chocolate sauce or champagne and lick it up.

Inside thigh

A big nerve centre where the skin is specially soft and receptive to every kind of touch: stroking, licking, tickling with feathers or trailing over with silky tassels. But save your treatment of this area till she's well warmed up and ready for you to travel on to the most erogenous zone of all.

Bottom

Kiss it, clutch it, press it, pamper it, stroke it and, if she likes that sort of thing, smack it—but not too hard. The bottom is soft and full of fatty tissue but also has plenty of nerve endings which makes it a very sexy place.

Back of knees

The pulse point at the back of her knees will flutter with ecstasy if you get to work with your lips and tongue on this incredibly sensitive spot. Many women dab their favourite scent on this area as a clue to you to get close—so if your nose leads you behind her knees, take the hint.

Shoulders

Use your thumbs to massage her shoulder muscles till you can feel her relax completely. If she shuts her eyes and puts her head back, you're really hitting the spot. Now titillate her senses by running your fingertips ever so lightly across her shoulder blades, circle them out as far as her armpits and back to the spine.

Breasts

Treat them to every tender touch you have at your fingertips: stroke and gently squeeze them, run your fingers backwards and forwards across the nipples till they harden and stand up with excitement; play with the nipples with fingers, lips, tongue—kiss, lick and suck them. And for a luxury taste treat, trickle a favourite tipple or chocolate sauce over them and lick it off.

Hands

The palms of her hands and insides of her wrists are incredibly sensitive areas which, if kissed and softly licked, can make her whole body tingle longingly at your touch. Suck softly on her fingers and thumbs and she should melt in your arms.

Toes

Kiss her toes and she'll know how much you want her. Her toes are full of nerve-ends which tell the brain you're turning her on with your loving lips and tongue. Massaging her feet with scented lotion is also a sensual treat and will help you find the right touch to tantalise rather than tickle.

And finally the G-spot

This is the one they used to argue about—whether it existed or whether its discoverer, gynaecologist Ernst Grafenberg, invented it. What now seems to be the case is that there *is* a pleasure zone where Grafenberg said there was—inside the vagina, on the front wall against the pubic bone—but researchers are divided over whether or not it is a female version of the prostate gland.

A caring and curious lover may find this pleasure point by feeling around with a finger—but it isn't worth agonising over. You can have a long and lusty, madly exciting sex life without ever getting to grips with the G-spot.

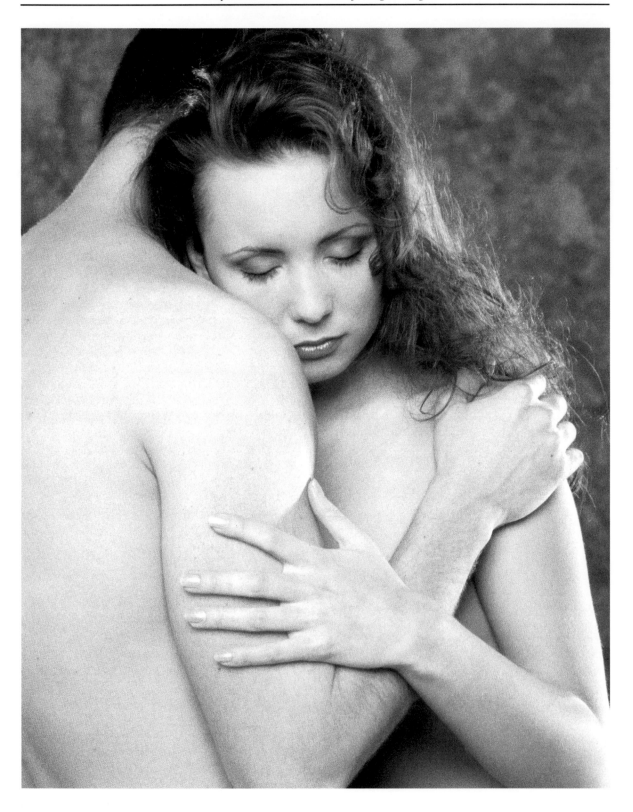

THE FIRST TIME
Starting a new relationship

The very first time you make love is a milestone which you will probably remember the rest of your life—whether it was sublime, so-so or something of a let-down. And it is often something of a let-down, after all the wondering, the wishing and comparing notes with friends. But remember, nobody's won Wimbledon the first time they've tried tennis. And, like tennis, sex gets better with practice.

Being nervous doesn't help anyone relax enough to enjoy this new and, we're constantly told, wonderful experience—and it wouldn't be human not to be nervous. We are all taught to expect so much—will the earth move? will the sky fill with fireworks?—that nothing could match the expectations.

The only certainty is, whatever happens, you will be glad it's over. Losing your virginity is something of a relief simply because at last you have an inkling of what everyone is talking about, what all those books, movies and songs are celebrating. So you won't die wondering. Phew.

David was a 19-year-old student when he found himself making love for the first time with his girlfriend, also a virgin till that night. He says: "It wasn't something we planned, we didn't decide we'd do it then. We were in my car and it just sort of happened. I was inside her and it wasn't like I'd imagined. I thought, 'So this is it. Oh well, it's a bit odd but I've got everything in the right place.'

"We did it again soon after and I then found out what was missing the first time: I hadn't ejaculated. The second time I did and as I felt it, I realised this was the crucial moment. I had never masturbated so I didn't know semen spurted out like it does, I imagined it just trickled.

"My girlfriend can't have known, either. She seemed happy enough and she never said anything."

Another first-timer, an 18-year-old medical student, was also a bit puzzled by his first full sexual performance: "I got my penis inside her and was lying on top thinking it was all a bit disappointing. I didn't know what to do next—nobody told me you had to move up and down."

For secretary Jackie, making love the first time was so unreal she felt as if she was watching herself experience it rather than actually doing it: "I'd read so many books about it that by the time it actually happened I felt like I was outside it waiting for the next step. The worst thing was I'd read that your breathing changed so I felt really self-conscious when I started panting. But I did enjoy it because it was with someone nice who really wanted me to have a good time."

So tonight's the night. Since the moment you met you've become closer and closer.

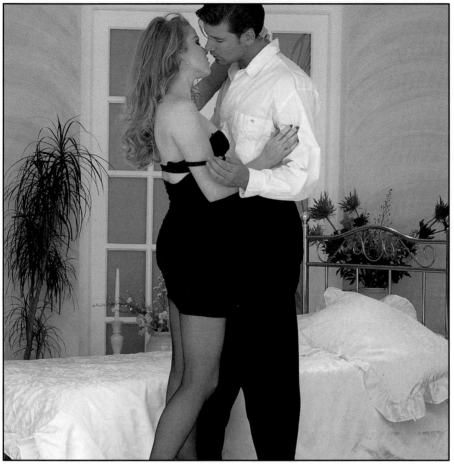

DO say: "I'd like to make love to you" or "Let's go to bed."

into bed together, here is how to make your first night performance more of a smash hit than a disastrous flop.... or at least a promising beginning to a lifetime's loving.

THE MOMENT

You long to leap on your partner and you're pretty sure the feeling's mutual. But how do you let them know you want to Do It Now? Grabbing and hoping for the best may give them such a fright they back off in confusion.

Making love happen when you want it is a better way of making it all-right-on-the-night than just getting carried away and getting on

And now you're about to stop being just good friends and become lovers.

Whether it's your first time ever or your first with a new partner, it can be equally nerve-wracking. What if you don't measure up? What if you realise after it's been a terrible mistake? *She* lay there like a dead jellyfish, *he* seemed to lose the urge at the critical moment; *he* had smelly feet, *she* had whiffy armpits. It can be sheer magic or desperately disappointing.

You can discover the best and worst things about someone once you slide between the sheets together. You also reveal the best and worst of yourself. And it's no consolation that others mostly share your fears.

So for all those lusty lovers about to jump

with it. If you're in control you can make sure there are no bad moments to mar the magic.

DO say: "I'd like to make love to you" or "Let's go to bed." It's the most flattering offer you can make anyone. It also makes your intentions clear so you don't get worked up to a state of wild abandon only to be told your partner hadn't reckoned on this being the right moment.

DON'T say: "What about it? Your place or mine?" You make it sound about as enticing as a game of darts.

DO invite him in for coffee, a nightcap or to see your movie posters—most men take this as code for a loving encounter.

DON'T do it unless you're sure your flatmates, your parents, your brothers and sisters are OUT. Or at least well out of the way. Being panicked into doing things too quickly will only add to any anxieties about performance on either side.

DO let your partner know if it is the very first time for you. There is no need to be embarrassed about this and it should ensure that, specially if they are quite experienced, they will be extra caring and considerate.

THE PLACE

DON'T opt for the back seat of the car, a park bench or anywhere else you might be disturbed. The danger of being caught might add thrills when you're long-time lovers but it can make your first time a fiasco. You'll be nervous enough without the fear of a policeman's torch or peeping Tom to interrupt you. Comfort and privacy are vital.

DO have low lighting, soft music, sweet smells of scented candles, pot pourri, incense. Anything that helps create a relaxed, dreamy mood will ease your inhibitions.

DON'T have bare light bulbs, bright overhead lights, pine or minty air freshener that makes the place smell like a public loo. It will tell your lover you're insensitive to your surroundings and may therefore be a less than sensitive lover.

DO have clean sheets, a tidy bedroom and clean bathroom. Making love in what smells like the locker room of a busy gym at the end of a hot day is enough to put anyone off their foreplay.

DON'T have a loo roll on the bedside table. It's a bit bog-

basic: tissues are less tacky. And try to hide your snaps of old girlfriends, boyfriends, exes or holiday frolics. Pin-ups of naked women in *his* bedroom will make *her* apprehensive and uncomfortable. Revealing polaroids of herself in basque and suspenders will immediately make *him* wonder who took them.

DO hide any sex manuals, videos or sex toys you may have—they may make your partner even more nervous about their performance.

DON'T try to inspire your lover with a pornographic movie. You want them to be turned on by *you*.

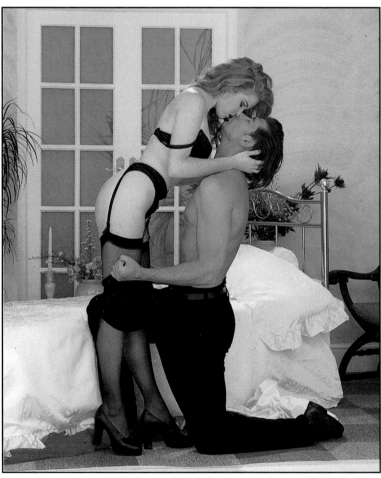

DO help your lover undress—it's all part of giving each other pleasure.

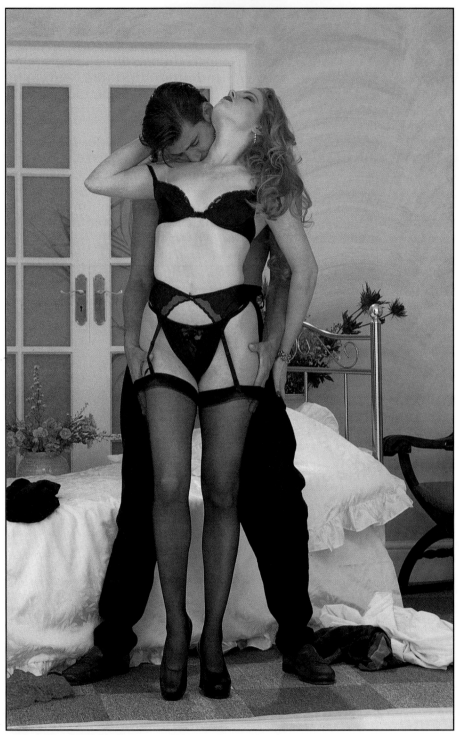

DO wear your laciest, wickedest bra, knickers, suspenders, stockings.

THE CLOTHES

Undressing in front of other people is always a bit embarrassing at first, unless you're a complete exhibitionist. Do you fling everything off regardless—or just enough to make sex possible? Do you undress each other or do it yourself? That's up to you. But you will feel most uncomfortable about sharing the intimate secrets of your underwear if it is in any way grubby, torn or tatty.

Clean underwear at all times is a must for him and her. But there are other garments that can kill passion as surely as saggy Y-fronts.

If you want to undress to thrill, you might think about the little details that make the difference.

FOR HER

DO wear silk, satin, velvet, fine cotton, lycra—which all feel irresistible to touch. DON'T wear anything that requires the delicate handiwork of a mastercraftsman to undo its fasteners. Or anything that fits like a glove and doesn't give easy access—like a bodystocking, camiknicker or other all-in-one. Unless he's very dainty-fingered he'll never be able to peel it off you without a struggle.

DO wear your laciest, wickedest bra, knickers, suspenders, stockings. Sports bras and leotards may look racy in the gym or changing room but they're a real challenge to remove by a lover with an attack of the fumbles.

DON'T put on the sort of undies you get from X-rated catalogues. Save them till you know his tastes. He may think you wear them all the time, on the off-chance.

FOR HIM

DON'T wear nylon socks, shirt or undies. If things get steamy, they can get that rotting vegetable smell.

DO wear tiny briefs or boxer shorts in whites or bright colours.

DON'T go for Y-fronts, G-strings or anything with saucy slogans like Keep It Up or Midnight Riser. She may think they're funny later but they're more likely to be off-putting at such an early stage.

DO get your socks off before you're starkers—they look silly on their own. And PLEASE, don't wear them to bed.

THE WORDS

"I love you" are the best words of all but only if you mean them and definitely not if you're only saying it to persuade someone to leap into bed with you.

The best love-talk at this stage is about what you're doing to each other and what you each most want.

"I really want to please you. Tell me what makes you feel good, what you'd most like me to do," is a good start. Every lover thrills to different touches and moves at a different pace. Finding out what gives your new partner ultimate pleasure, then trying to give it, is the sign of a skilled and caring lover. But you don't have to have sampled dozens of lovers to do this, you just need to be sexually well-educated—and to enjoy giving.

We all worry about saying the wrong thing. Or about saying anything at all. Not everyone has a way with words—silence is preferable to coming out with any of the following:

"I don't do this with everyone."

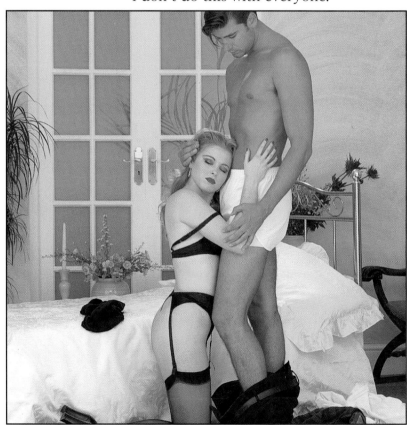

For him—DO wear tiny briefs or boxer shorts in whites or bright colours.

"Was it good for you?
"Will you still respect me in the morning?"
"I've never seen one like that before"
"Is that it?"
"Ouch, get off, you're hurting."
"I've never done it like this before"
"Not like that, like this"
"I think I need another glass of wine"
"I think I've had too much to drink"
"What's that funny smell?"
"What's that funny noise?"
"Have you finished yet?"

THE MOVES

Anything goes as long as you both enjoy it, the experts say. But there are some moves that are almost always a mistake the first time around.

DON'T grab straight for the sexy bits, even if you are in a hurry. *Everyone* likes the fun of foreplay first and sex will be better as a result.

DO wait till her sex organs are moist enough to be entered comfortably. If her body is ready for love, there is more chance of it being a pleasurable experience for both of you.

DON'T worry if he starts to lose his erection and go limp. First-time sex is daunting for everyone but a man's nervousness can show in a more obvious way than a woman's. Help by gently massaging him back to hardness.

DO help your lover undress—it's all part of giving each other pleasure. But don't go at it like a chocoholic ripping the wrapper off a Mars bar. Slow is sexier this time, when you're both trying to sense your new partner's likes and dislikes.

DON'T hide in the bathroom or in the dark while you undress—it'll make your lover think you're trying to conceal something

DO have lots of kisses and cuddles afterwards to make your mate feel wanted. Women need to feel their partner cares, men need to feel their partner is satisfied. If a woman doesn't have an orgasm the first time, that's not at all unusual.

DON'T jump up straight afterwards and start pulling your clothes on

DO go to sleep in each other's arms—even if one of you does have to go home afterwards

DON'T just happen to have a change of clothing and your toilet things with you. It might seem too ready for anything—with anyone.

DO have a spare pair of clean knickers or underpants and a travelling tooth-brush. They'll always make you feel fresh.

THE MUSTS

Condoms may seem unromantic and unduly prepared—but they're a must for making love with a new mate as they are the surest protection against the risk of sexually transmitted diseases, as well as helping avoid an unwanted pregnancy.

So do have a pack in your handbag or pocket. If you're a woman, don't be daft enough to think you'll look cheap by doing so. Wise, sensible, intelligent and responsible are more appropriate words for condom-carrying than cheap. It is also the sign of a thoughtful lover not to rely on your partner to have some handy. You can get them free at any Family Planning Clinic, so there's no excuse.

Waiting till you're both aroused is not the best moment to whisper, 'Had we better use a condom?' Try to get it straight between you so that you have protection at hand before you're too excited to care. Some people are foolishly not as careful as others about insisting on safe sex and it would be sad to clash on this issue at an emotionally tender time. Try to bring up the subject beforehand to establish how each of you feels, so you can agree on what to do about contraception and keeping safe from AIDS.

And finally, if you find yourself in a sex shop buying condoms, it is probably better to have them in ordinary transparent skin tones the first time and not lurid colours. A new partner may also be put off by ones with knobs, bumps, funny faces or exotic flavours. Save them for when you want to try something new and daring with a tried and trusted partner.

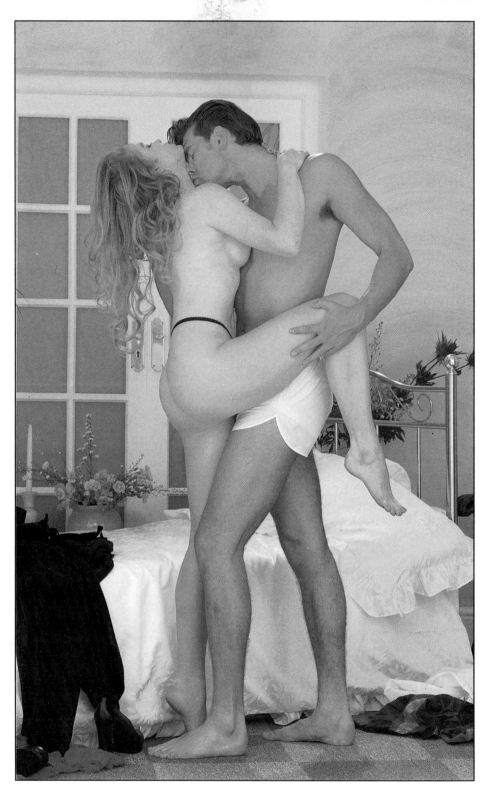

Everyone likes the fun of foreplay first and sex will be better as a result.

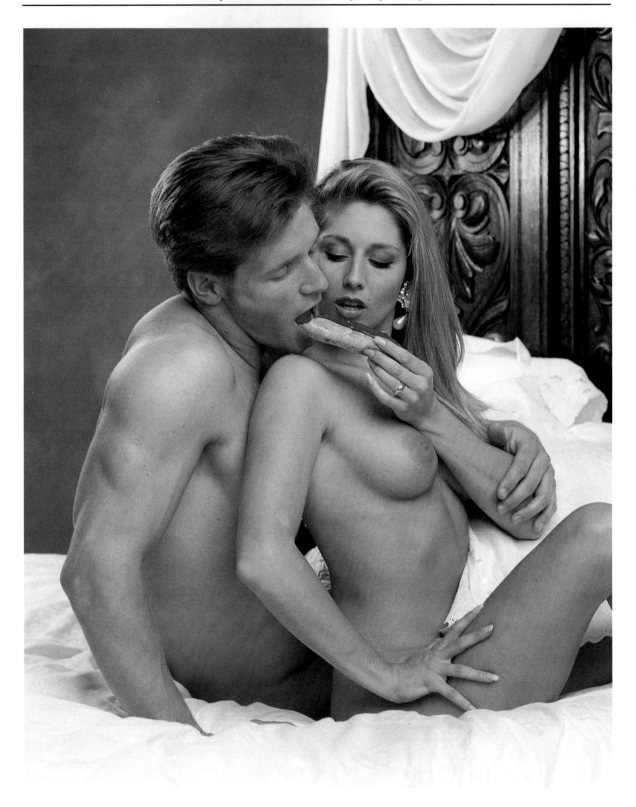

FOREPLAY
Love that lasts all day

When you ask what men and women want from sex, men usually say "More sex" and women say "More foreplay." In what seems like an unfair trick of fate, men and women are in different time-zones when it comes to getting the urge to jump on each other. A man can often just look at a woman and feel the stirrings of lust and longing that need to be gratified. A woman usually takes longer to reach a state of excitement that has her tearing at her man. Scientists say this is nature's way of keeping the population down—if women were as randy as men they would lose their power to choose a mate, based on his ability to protect and provide.

But it is a wild exaggeration to say that men are on permanent stand-by for sex at every opportunity while women have to be slowly wooed, stroked and teased to the point of passion. Men like to be lovingly worked up to a lather of excitement as well. They also like to be told, not necessarily in words, that they are wanted, desired and longed for.

Women have put so much pressure on men to perform that the stress of satisfying *her* frequently loses him his impetus. Where women used to excuse themselves from sex with real or imaginary headaches, now men have joined the race for the aspirin.

The trouble with foreplay is that it's got more like a game of badminton or tennis than a loving encounter between two people: warm up by kissing for two minutes, his hand goes for her breast, her hand reaches for his rear. Take turns to touch—pat, pat, tit for tat—till you're both vaguely convinced the other is ready. Then go for the big serve and try to smash and volley your way to ecstasy.

But foreplay is not just a series of strokes guaranteed to raise your partner's temperature and enthusiasm. It can be anything from thoughtful gestures, helpful deeds and loving words spoken long before you lay a finger on each other. When women complain of lack of foreplay what they so often say is that, out of the blue, they are confronted by a hairy hand reaching into their blouse or under their skirt. No smooching, no darling-you're-driving-me crazy-with-lust, no hand-holding while you watch telly. He just homes in on the basics.

Now, sometimes that's what's wanted. If you've had a good night out together—or perhaps haven't seen each other for a week—you may well want to pounce on each other like wildcats as soon as your front door's shut. But probably most of the time you will need a more leisurely warm up to love.

The tricky thing about women is the unpredictability of their bodies—one day the most arousing thing a man can do is fondle and squeeze and kiss and nibble their breasts. And another day those breasts will be a no-go area. So a man has to feel his way sensitively and slowly.

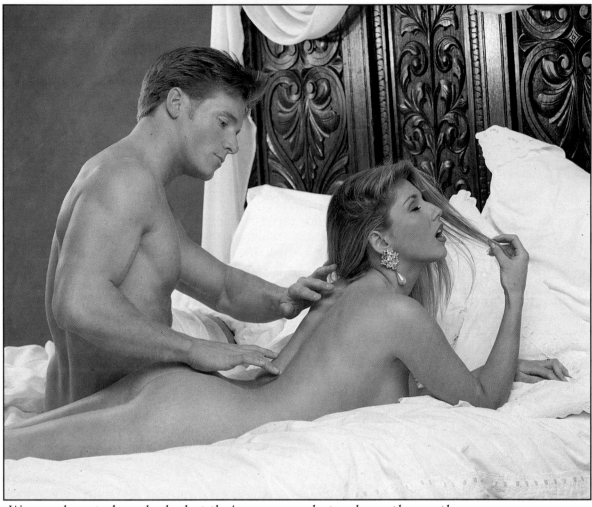

Women love to be asked what their man can do to please them—they know then that he wants to please them.

The best favour he can do the woman he loves is probably the most difficult: ask her what she wants. Men often can't bring themselves to do this because they feel they're supposed to know their way round every millimetre of a woman's body. But women love to be asked what their man can do to please them—they know then that he *wants* to please them.

The one thing a man *can* be sure of, the more time he spends talking to her, sharing his thoughts, including her in his life, telling her he loves her, giving her a kiss or squeeze for no reason other than affec-

tion—at any time of day or night—the more thrilled she will be when he is stirred by animal passion.

But women should be aware that men also like to feel loved and cared for at other times than moments of lust. *He* doesn't enjoy it when she grabs straight for the contents of his boxer shorts, either.

FOREPLAY IS NOT ONLY SEXY STROKES AND SQUEEZES BUT ALSO:
• Phoning your loved one just to let them know you were thinking about them and it made you feel all warm and randy

- A gentle peck on the cheek when they're mending the washing machine or making the dinner
- Telling her she looks better than Sharon Stone
- Telling him you love the feel of his muscles
- Buying a silly, inexpensive present because you know it's something they want
- Giving your lover a neck massage while they tell you the troubles of their day
- Saying "I love you" at any time
- A candlelit dinner with time to talk
- Snuggling up beside them and reading a book while they study or do the work they brought home
- Writing a love poem for them
- Telling each other every little thing you'd like to do to give their body pleasure
- Washing your partner's hair and drying it for them
- Manicuring their nails or massaging their feet with cooling foot lotion

TEASE HIM TO PLEASE HIM
Though you may not always be aware of it, every time you take your clothes off your man is watching. Men are visually-stimulated animals who get very excited when they see something they like.

If you undress in the dark or behind the bathroom door you'll not only be depriving your man but giving him a sign that says no to sex.

On the other hand, the way you dress will tell him whether you are geared up for bedtime frolics.

For instance, you may think that slinky black dress with all the buttons down one side will make his tongue hang out with longing for what's underneath.

But he will just think it looks like hard work fiddling with all those buttons and worry that he might lose the urge while he fiddles.

But his eyes will light up at the sight of the demure white shift with the zip down the back—he knows he can undress you in seconds with one hand while he caresses you intimately with the other.

Some men are all thumbs when it comes to unhooking the most basic of bras. But if you wear one that fastens in the front at least he can see what he's doing while fondling your breasts at the same time. Your man will get to know that if you're wearing one of these, his handiwork will be welcome. But if you're all caught up in a stretchy, strappy sports bra with no fasteners at all, it's just not his night.

Silky bare legs uncovered by tights or stockings are a definite come-on: no problems with snagging her best 7-deniers in the height of passion.

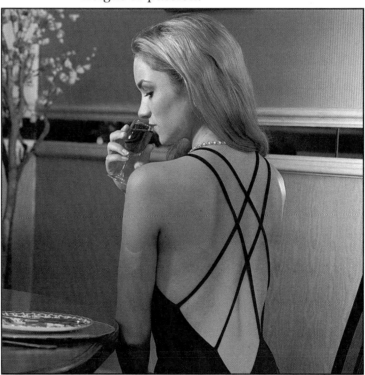

That slinky black dress may make him think it looks like hard work fiddling to remove it.

A see-through top that's just sheer enough to suggest you're *probably* bra-less is irresistible and he won't be able to tear his eyes away till he's sure. He may even have to use his hands to find out—and that's the idea, isn't it?

The sort of softly clinging dress that covers you up while revealing every goose-bump is guaranteed to drive your man crazy—wondering whether or not you're wearing knickers (you wouldn't want the dreaded Visible Pantie Line, would you?)

Kicking off your shoes and dancing bare-foot says you're feeling wild and wanton—specially if you're stroking his leg with your bare toes while you're smooching.

Seeing a part of you he's not meant to see at that moment will really tickle your man's fancy. So when you head for the bathroom, try letting your bath-robe fall to the floor a split second before closing the door, giving him an intimate glimpse of nakedness. Or let the towel round your body slip down as you stand before the mirror drying your hair.

He will love to watch you getting out of

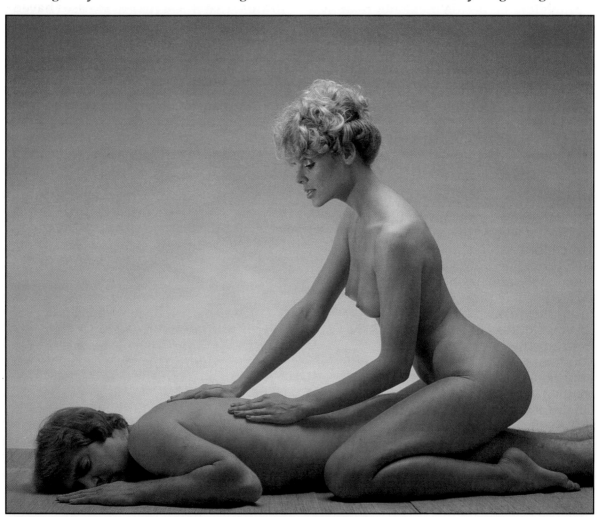

Massage is the greatest treat and can be a long, luxurious turn-on which makes the receiver feel deliciously spoiled, pampered and utterly relaxed.

your working day clothes and into something loose for an evening at home. But not if you tear them off as if they're on fire.

Do it slowly, starting by unfastening your skirt, dress or trousers which you let drop to the floor and step out of it. Next, slowly unbutton your top and peel it off so you're left in just your undies and high heels.

Put one foot on the edge of a chair or the bed while you ease off a stocking, replacing the shoe. Switch feet to remove the other stocking.

Run your hands slowly up and down your body before s-l-o-w-l-y removing your bra. Then your knickers. Let him feast his eyes before slipping into something silky—or not. You may now both be so hungry for a sexy starter that you can't wait till dinner time.

And finally, if you want to give him the kind of sexy surprise he may only have thought happened in fantasy, plan ahead to make his dream come true.

Get the most frivolous, sexy basque or bra-and-suspenders set and slip them in your bag on a night out. Just before you head for home, slip into the nearest Ladies and swap your dress for your undies so they are all you're wearing under your coat.

As he closes the front door behind you, let your coat slip to the floor and give him an eyeful. It will make his night—whatever you do afterwards.

IN THE MOOD?

Knowing when your mate is in the mood for love can be as tricky as mind-reading or as easy as ABC—as long as you can crack their love-code.

Many couples who have been together a long time use their own very personal, often quirky, signals to let each other know when tonight's the night.

Some lovers reveal their secret signs:

"When my wife strips down to nothing but her necklace, I know she's feeling randy. If she takes her necklace off before bed, I know sex might be off as well."

"I wear his favourite flimsy night-dress and let him see me squirting perfume behind my ears—and my knees."

"My husband takes his clothes off then wanders round singing 'I'm in the nude for love.'"

"When my wife wears a dress zipped up the front or back, I know my chances of nookie are high. If she's in jeans and a sweater, it's unpromising."

"If my husband shaves at night instead of in the morning I know he's got his mind on fun and games at bedtime. In case I haven't noticed he sometimes takes my hand, places it on his cheek and says, 'Smooth as a baby's bottom?'"

"When my wife takes my hand and starts sucking on my little finger I know it's time to carry her off to the bedroom."

"If he leaves the landing light on when we go to bed I know he's in the mood because he likes to see what he's doing. We don't like to make love with the bright bedroom light on."

"If he says he can't be bothered staying up for Match of the Day and then spends a long time splashing round in the bathroom I know he's getting ready for love."

"She takes her shoes off and walks round barefoot on her toes. Then she sits near me and rests her feet on my knees so I can massage them. That's her signal."

"When he suggests we take our coffee and liqueurs up to bed after a good dinner, I know what's coming next."

FEELING THE WAY

Good foreplay is all about giving each other what you want and is what makes a good lover.

Selfish and lazy lovers aren't bothered enough to find out what makes a partner tremble with excitement. As long as they are warming to a lover's touch they are happy to lie back and be treated.

For many, foreplay is the best part of sex:

the slow build-up of physical excitement, the holding back to make the thrills of arousal go on and on, the novelty of discovering new ways to excite your mate.

START SLOWLY is the message most women and many men would like to get across. And try to save the best till last. As Danni, 23, puts it: "Some men are so anxious to get straight to the clitoris as if it was some kind of starter button. But I need to be touched all over my body before getting to that. I have to be really aroused by being very gently stroked and caressed till my skin is all warm and tingling and I'm aching for him to touch me down there."

Ian, 29, says: "Women say men want to progress too quickly but they're the ones who often grab straight for your goolies. Some of them think they're the only sexy part a man has."

TALKING about sex and each other's preferences is a big turn-on, specially for women. A man who spends time getting to know what they want is stimulating their sexiest part—the brain.

Ellie, 32, says: "When he tells me he wants to taste every part of me with his tongue or asks how I feel about having my toes kissed or nipples sucked, it makes me feel incredibly excited."

HUGS AND CUDDLES make both him and her feel wanted and safe, a feeling essential to good loving. Being relaxed in your lover's arms makes you feel wanted for yourself and not just as a sex object.

Mary, 40, says: "I want to feel loved, above all. Lusted after is nice but only if you can feel waves of affection enveloping you. The loving relationship is what matters most to me."

Ross, 38, says: "Having her wrapped round me like a kitten, all soft and purring, makes me feel so protective and trusted. I melt."

MASSAGE is the greatest treat and can be a long, luxurious turn-on which makes the receiver feel deliciously spoiled, pampered and utterly relaxed. A good top-to-toe massage with scented body oil should take about an hour and make your partner feel both soothed and sexy. If she's feeling frazzled or he's had a hard day, it's the perfect way to stroke away tension and prepare for love.

For John, 34, massage proved the answer to satisfying lovemaking with wife Alison: "Sometimes I felt I was rushing her or that she was tired and often not in the mood. It was frustrating for both of us. Then one evening I decided to surprise her by offering a massage with some special herby body oil that's supposed to make you feel relaxed and refreshed. She loved it and so did I— specially the wonderful, totally exhausting sex we had afterwards."

SURPRISES add sparkle to sex which can get routine and predictable when a couple has been together a long time. If you always make love at the same time of day, same days of the week, same position, same place—try changing the details. Make love early in the morning before work; Saturday afternoon instead of going to the supermarket; do it in your work clothes as soon as you get home; do it on the kitchen floor instead of in the bedroom. Variety is the spice of sex.

Josie, 29, says: "We were in a bit of a rut sexwise. Never any time, always rushing about and not thinking of each other enough. I thought if it went on like that there wasn't much point being together. So I started thinking about sex more, setting the scene.

"I'd do things like one night on the way back from work I started groping Mike in the car till he had to pull over. We went off down a leafy lane and parked in a cul-de-sac where we made love like teenagers. He was amazed. He thought I'd gone crazy or taken a love potion or something. Now we do daft things like that often."

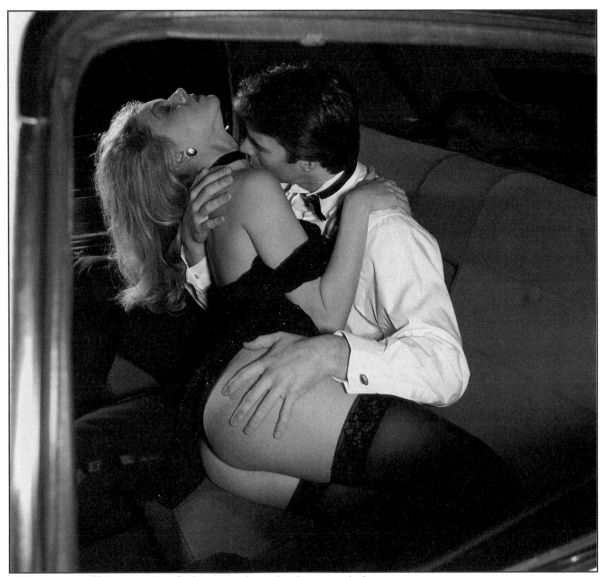

*"We went off down a leafy lane and parked in a cul-de-sac
where we made love like teenagers."*

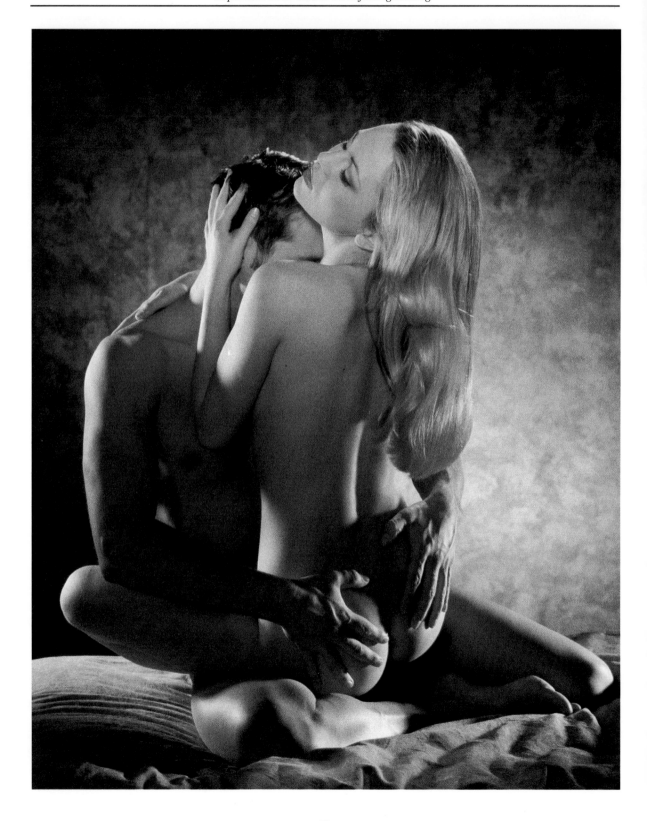

THE POSITION IS THIS
Sexual positions—a consumer guide

Lying down, sitting up, sideways, on all fours or on one leg, you can enjoy sex every which way. As long as the genitals lock into each other—or even get their excitement from other parts of a lover's body—that's sexual intercourse. The variations are seemingly endless, as any browse through the Kama Sutra will tell you. Work your way through that lot and you won't be able to walk for a month. But is that what you want? Probably not.

After you've tried a few of the more exotic sexual gymnastics which have left you nursing bruises, pulled muscles and wondering why you bothered, you have probably settled happily back into the missionary position. That's the one where *he* lies on top and *she* lies under him with her legs apart—basic, comfortable and used by most couples at least some of the time.

It's thought by some to be very boring and unimaginative but that probably has more to do with its name than the activity itself. One does not imagine missionaries mating with a wild lack of inhibition. But in fact this perfectly useful, practical position, which has made the earth shake on its axis since kingdom come, was not invented by those who took Christianity to primitive parts of the globe. It got its name when Polynesian natives in the South Pacific noticed that the missionaries' way of making love was different from their own. The natives found this both curious and funny.

But that is probably nothing compared with the missionaries' reaction to the Polynesian way of sex—the man squatted on the ground and the woman lay on her back, wriggling towards him till she could hang her thighs over his and ease his erect penis into her vagina. Gobsmacked would be more like it. Wonder how many of them went away and tried it?

Positions are a matter of personal choice depending on your attitude to sex, your athleticism, your adventurousness—and whatever takes your fancy at the time. Doing it standing up against a tree may not have a lot going for it in that it's hard to get maximum pleasure while keeping your balance and keeping watch against prying eyes. But if you happen to be overcome by friskiness while walking in the park, the tree position's the one you'll choose. If you're the sort of feminist who snarls when a man opens a door for you, you may refuse to have sex lying on your back with a man on top, pinning you to the bed or floor. If you're Macho Mickey who feels good only when he's ravishing a woman in an apron and rubber gloves pinned against her kitchen sink, you won't want her sitting astride your prone torso riding you like a bucking bronco.

So every position has its fans and its critics. With that in mind, here's how to decide what goes where when you're stripped for action and so steamed up you can't tell your thigh from your thumbs.

1. Him on Top, Her Flat on her Back.
With his legs between hers, this is the most basic missionary position and there is no mystery about its popularity. Because of the angle at which the man enters the woman, it gives a lot of pleasure to both while looking into each other's eyes, feeling the length of each other's body pressing close, being able to kiss and whisper loving words all at the same time. Humans are the only animals who make love facing each other—the others all do it from the rear—and this is the most close and intimate of all lovemaking positions. So don't knock it.

It may not be so great, however, if a man is huge and a woman so slender she is crushed by his weight. Unless the woman is strong enough to move her hips up and down along with the pelvic thrusts of her lover—done easily if she plants her feet down just in front of her bottom and pushes up-wards—it can be a bit of a one-sided ma-noeuvre.

2. Him on Top, Her Legs Wrapped Round His Waist. He can thrust deeper inside her while she hangs on tight with her legs, clenching his hips against hers with her crossed ankles. A bit more energetic than the basic version, with more activity on her part and more rewarding for him, being wrapped in what amounts to an all-over hug. The stronger her thighs, the more thrilling for both. And for women who like to fight back rather than just lie there, this one's good for morale. Not a position for prolonged loving, but great for a strong and speedy climax.

3. Him on Top, Her Legs Over His Shoulders. This position may be the ori-gin of the definition of foreplay Down Un-der: "Brace yourself, Raelene." Because that's about all the woman can do in this situa-

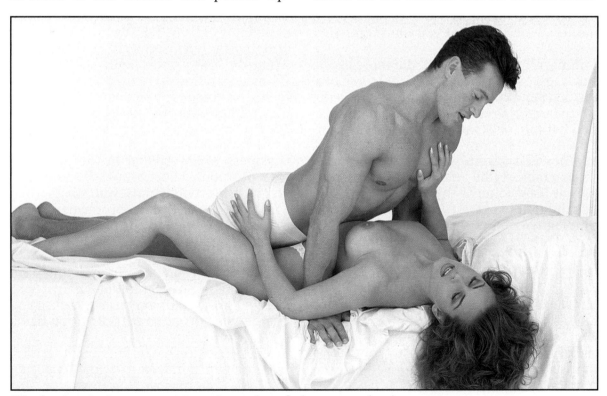

The basic missionary position gives a lot of pleasure to both, while looking into each other's eyes.

tion. The penetration of the penis is very deep which can give enormous pleasure to both partners. But hugging, kissing, caressing are fairly much out of the question since he has to keep his balance supported by his outstretched arms and she can't reach many parts of him to add to his enjoyment. If you're the kind of woman who doesn't like to feel dominated by a man, you may not feel thrilled by this position.

4. Him on his Side, Her Legs Over His Hips. You probably wouldn't start off with this position but get to it after hugging and kissing while both are lying on their side, his penis clamped between her upper thighs. Once she has manoeuvred into the legs-over position so he can penetrate her, she will be lying on her back at right angles to him. It may not seem much fun for him but she can get a lot of excitement from the fact that he has both arms free to fondle her

nearest breast as well as her clitoris. He can also watch her face to see the effect his lovemaking is having. And she can squeeze his testicles and stroke the base of his penis. This can be a good way to make love during pregnancy—but you have to save kissing till afterwards.

5. Him On His Back, Her on Top Lying Down. Physically great for both, as long as neither has attitude problems over who is on top. It's great for him because she can place herself on his penis so it goes in deeply; because his hands are free to caress her breasts; because he can kiss her breasts or her lips; because he can stroke her bottom and hold her tightly to him by clutching her buttocks; because he can gaze into her eyes. It is great for her for all the reasons listed already—plus the fact she doesn't have his weight pressing down on her. Quite good during pregnancy for this

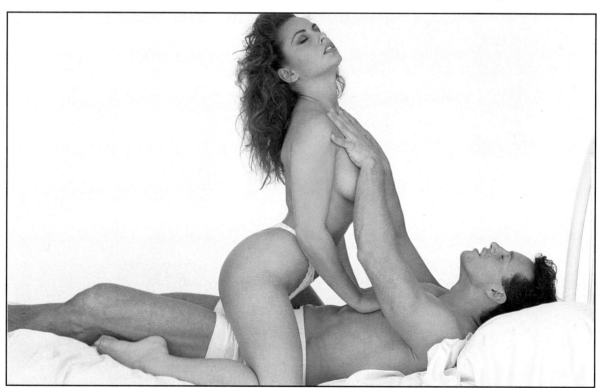

Him on his back, her on top kneeling, gives even better and deeper penetration. Both partners can stroke and squeeze each other's nipples.

reason also. But for all the women who enjoy the comfort and freedom of being on top, there are as many others who would rather their man felt dominant.

6. Him on His Back, Her on Top Kneeling. Even better and deeper penetration than the previous position with the added attraction, for her, of being able to grind her pubic bone against his for extra stimulation to the clitoris. He or she can also reach the clitoris easily with their fingers. Both partners can stroke and squeeze each other's nipples and she can reach behind her and hold his testicles. For him, there is the increased pleasure to be had

from being able to see not only her face but most of her body and their combined sexual activity—a major turn-on for the male which is not particularly shared by the female.

7. Him on His Back, Her Squatting on Top. Expect maximum penetration, which is brilliant for both as long as there is no significant size discrepancy—that is, if he is outstandingly well-endowed length-wise this position may be extremely uncomfortable for her. His penis pressing against the uterus could hurt—but a woman in this position can control the depth of penetration so there shouldn't be a problem. It is not one of the cuddly, affectionate posi-

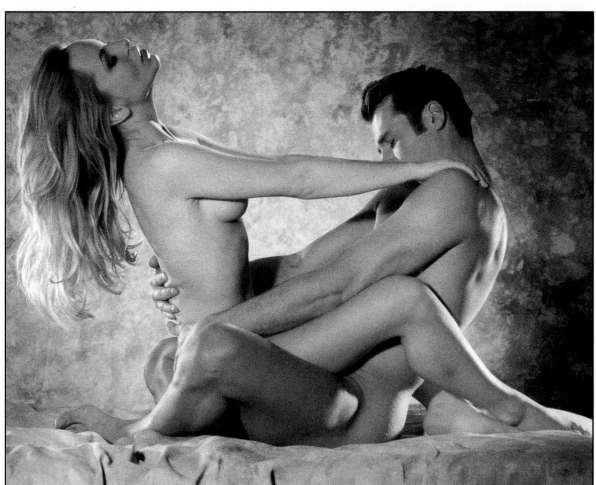

Him sitting, legs in front, her sitting facing him, legs over his—a great position if you're feeling wide awake and eager for maximum stimulation.

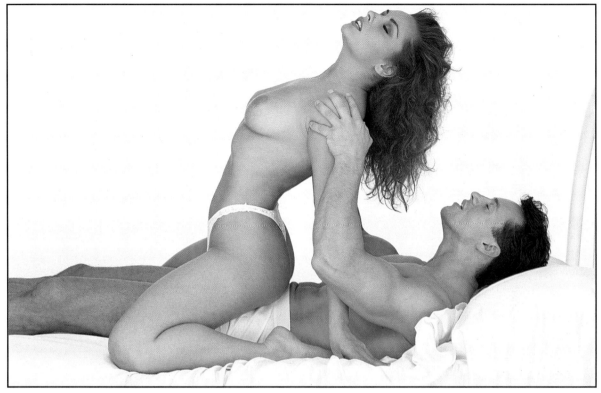

Him lying, her kneeling on top with her back to him. You wouldn't do this on your first night with a new lover, but as a new trick with an old lover it is a good variation.

tions, however, so it's likely to leave you feeling you've had sex rather than made love. Fine for those times when you're so randy you want to do it every which way. Not so good when you want to feel close.

8. Him Lying, Her Kneeling on Top with Her Back To Him. You wouldn't do this as an early move in a passion session or on your first night with a new lover, as it might seem rudely impersonal. Can she not stand the sight of his face? Is he trying to tell her something about her looks? But as a new trick with an old lover it is a good variation that gives a new slant on the angle of the penis—which won't find its own way into the vagina without a helping hand. For both partners this is both comfortable and full of rousing sensations to make sex sizzle. If she is very supple, an acrobatic variation is for her to lower herself backwards till she lies

along his body. He can then increase her excitement by stroking her clitoris. This position should really hit the G-spot.

9. Him Sitting, Legs in Front. Her Sitting Facing Him, Legs Over His. She will have to raise herself enough to be able to lead his penis to the entrance of her vagina, before lowering herself so he is comfortably inside her. A great position if you're feeling wide awake and eager for maximum stimulation (if you're feeling like warm, dozy lovemaking with minimum effort, forget it). Sitting opposite each other like this, you can stroke each other's hair and face, kiss and suck each other's fingers, hug each other tight, gently play with each other's breasts, rock backwards and forwards so you really feel the depth of penetration possible in this position.

10. Him on His Back, Her on her Back On Top. Comfortable for him, easy for her, since both are lying flat on their back. It does make it more exciting, though, if she arches her back for deeper thrusting of the penis inside her. If he raises his knees between her legs, resting his feet on the bed, it can make things easier as well, by giving her support. This is really a variation of what is known as the 'spoons' position, where the couple lie on their side facing the same way with his knees tucked into the back of her thighs. But while the spoons position makes a woman feel warm and protected, this version is a bit more abandoned and adventurous, with her legs flung apart instead of being loosely together.

11. Him Sitting Cross-Legged. Her Lying Back, Legs Round his Waist. She has to climb onto his lap, guiding his penis inside her, before wrapping her legs round him and linking her ankles. Then she holds his hands and lets him lower her slowly back till she is lying down. Phew, it takes a bit of organising but many women find the ecstasy that results is worth the gymnastic effort. It is fun for him, too, as long as he is agile enough to support her on his knees—though he could make it easier on himself by simply sitting

with his knees apart and letting her rest on his feet. He can caress her clitoris and feast his eyes on most of her body at the same time.

12. Her on All Fours, Him Kneeling Behind. The doggy position sounds beastly but is voted a hit with both sexes. It is easy for the man to slide his penis into his lover's vagina from behind and the angle of penetration gives a lot of pleasure without requiring acrobatics or strength. The woman can do very little to give her partner extra pleasure except push back against him as he thrusts. But he can reach her genitals with his fingers and fondle her hips, bottom and tummy. If she drops to her elbows and puts her head down, she and her mate can get even deeper satisfaction.

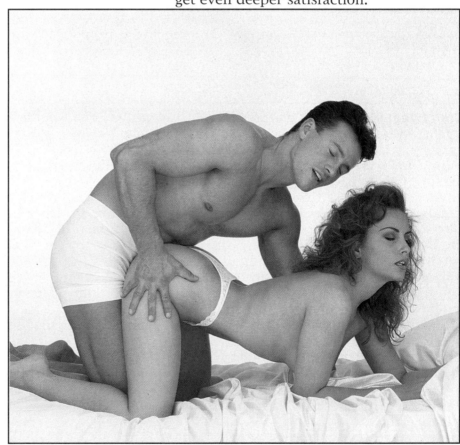

Her on all fours, him kneeling behind—sounds beastly but is voted a hit with both sexes.

13. Her on Her Stomach, Him on Top. If she's feeling too lazy for the last position, by rolling onto her stomach with her legs apart she can let her partner enter from behind. Once again, she can't caress him and can't see his face. But his hands are freer to roam round to her breasts and clitoris and he can kiss the back of her neck, round her ears—and her mouth, if she twists her head around.

14. Her Face Down, Resting on Her Elbows. Him Kneeling Behind, Holding Up Her Thighs. This is the grown-up version of what you did in the wheelbarrow race as a child. Sort of. In this position, she can do absolutely nothing except let him thrust away, doing all the work. Plenty of women may have problems with this one as they feel it's a demeaning posture. It is also about as impersonal as sex can get—which no doubt suits some less affectionate lovers.

15. Her on Her Back, Him Kneeling, Holding Up Her Thighs. Same as above, only her position is reversed so you can see each other's faces and what's going on between you. A definite improvement in intimacy terms. Can feel pretty raunchy and it's easy for him to move to the standard missionary position to finish.

16. Him Behind Her, Both on Their Side. This is the spoons position, famously comfortable for pregnant women and very cuddly in a big-man-protects-little-woman sort of way. There's no pressure on anybody to perform when in this position, you can both relax and enjoy yourselves. He can fondle her all over from behind and she can reach back and play with his sexiest bits. It's possible to kiss as well and the rear-entry penetration of the vagina is easy and pretty satisfying. A not very taxing but useful and usually pleasant experience.

17. Him on a Chair, Her on His Lap. It's a different angle, it's a change, it's an easy position for him, being supported by the chair. And whether she sits astride and facing him, with her back to him or even

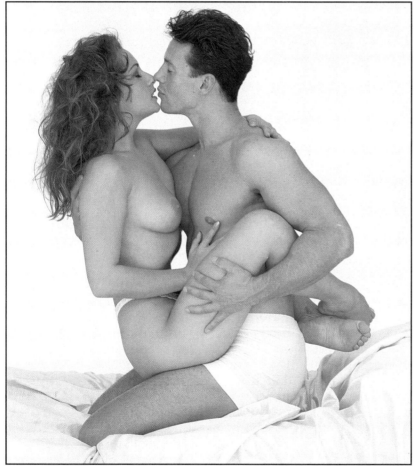

Him sitting cross-legged. Her lying back, legs round his waist. She has to climb onto his lap, before wrapping her legs round him and linking her ankles. Then she holds his hands and lets him lower her slowly back.

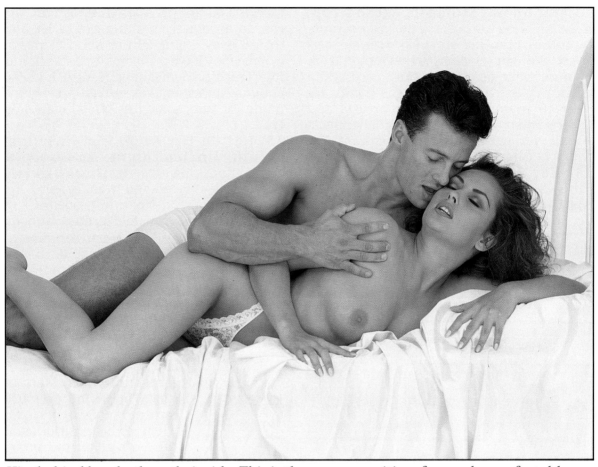

Him behind her, both on their side. This is the spoons position, famously comfortable for pregnant women and very cuddly in a big-man-protects-little-woman sort of way.

sideways, a lot of handiwork is possible for both partners. With all hands free and all feet on the ground, this is one position that enables loving fingers to reach the parts other positions don't allow. Penetration is deepish, you can see each other and kiss and cuddle. This one is no doubt popular among lovers who do it at the office.

18. Her Lying on Bed or Table, Him Standing. She lies on her back with her bottom near the edge of the bed or table. He stands between her open thighs, which he hangs onto with both hands, and enters her—probably with a helping hand from her. It is relaxing for her if she's on a bed—less comfortable but more thrilling if it's

the kitchen or dining table on which she's spreadeagled. There's not much chance of fondling—he's gripping her thighs and she's too far back to reach him—but both can see the look of ecstasy on each other's faces and the point where he enters her body.

19. Both Standing, Her with One Leg Round Him. Sex is not easy standing up—but it's usually fun as it tends to take place in daring locations: parks, shop doorways, broom cupboards. It helps if she leans against the wall (or tree) and it's easier for couples of near-equal height. If she can wrap one leg around him it will help hold them together—the thrusting action of intercourse isn't easy in this position. This is not one for comfort or orgasmic quality but good for spontaneous quickies when the mood takes you.

20. Him Sitting, Her Lying, Each Holding the Other's Feet. He sits with his legs apart, knees slightly raised. She lies on her back, puts her legs over his thighs and wriggles into position so that he can enter her. He then clasps her with the palms of his hands against the soles of her feet and she hangs onto the soles of his feet as well. Because the hands and feet are such sensitive erogenous zones this position can feel extremely erotic—and different. Definitely worth a try when you're feeling experimental.

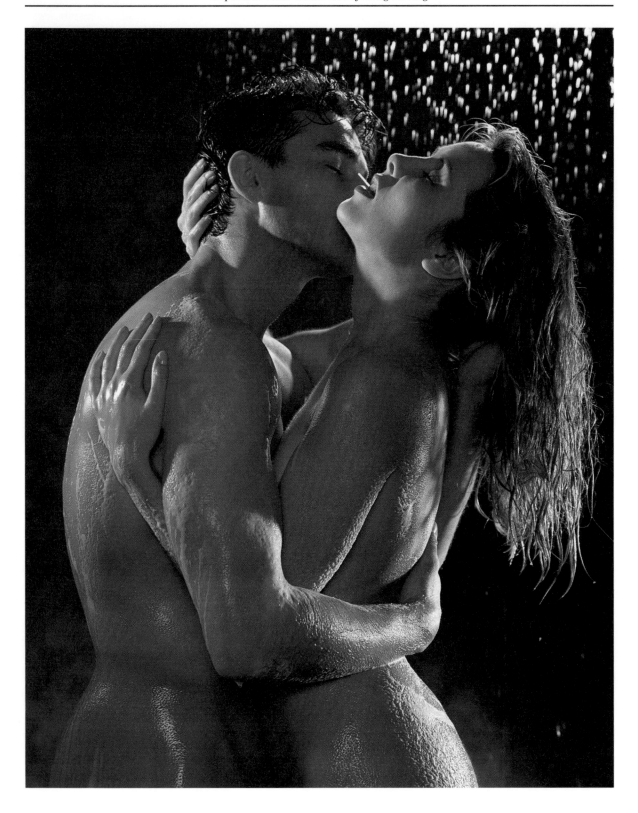

WHERE TO DO IT

Bedrooms, bathrooms, bike sheds and back seats

Fun lovers with a spirit of adventure like to notch up new locations for lovemaking whenever they get the chance. The challenge of a passionate encounter in a less than private place is always irresistible to them. For while the security of your own bedroom is perfect for the kind of marathon love-in enjoyed by newlyweds and others in the white-hot stages of early love, more dangerous situations offer excitement to those wanting to spice up a longstanding relationship.

There must be few places in the world where couples have not made love. As long as there is room for two people to lock together in a loving embrace, it can be done. All you need is to keep a crafty eye out for places which might appeal to you and your lover as a change of scene from the room in which you sleep every night.

Having said that, of the six million people making love as you read this, the majority will be doing it in a bedroom.

When we're having our early sexual experiences, fumbling in cars, in bus shelters, behind the bike sheds and on park benches, all we wish is that we could dive into a big, soft, warm bed and enjoy each other's bodies in privacy and comfort. But there are the usual problems of smuggling each other past parents and families to reach our own little rooms. A snog on the living room sofa is about as far as many of us get to loving in comfort at that stage, with all the worry of being interrupted or heard. The other most

popular petting place is probably on or under the pile of coats flung on a spare bed by guests at a party. The same problems apply. No wonder we cling to our bedrooms as havens from the world once we become independent adults.

But, intimate and precious as this space is to us, many don't make the most of it as a sensuous setting for love. Yet women, especially, are susceptible to romantic surroundings, so lovemaking will certainly be enhanced by a bedroom tailored to your sexiest needs and whims. When we spend about a third of our lives in bed, it seems madness not to make it as blissful a place as possible. Why not a baby fridge for lovers' sips and snacks? Why not a remote-control stereo?

But first things first. The bed doesn't have to be the ornately carved and curtained four-poster of honeymooners' dreams but it should be the best you can afford. Cheap beds are less likely to stand the strain of enthusiastic mattress-pounding and can collapse under the pressure. Also, they can be bad for your back—and there's nothing worse for your sex life than a dodgy back.

Sheets are a matter of personal taste—some like the crisp freshness of white cotton while others prefer the silky feel and sexy look of black satin. It has to be said that nylon sheets can get sweaty in the heat of passion and that flannelette may remind you of your granny and the smell of Vick's. It's up to you—the only must is that they should always be clean and sweet-smelling. And dousing dirty sheets with a splash of aftershave or cologne will not boost their fragrance-rating.

Lighting can be more of a passion-killer than grey underpants, if it is both harsh and shining down from the ceiling. It is thought that those who like making love

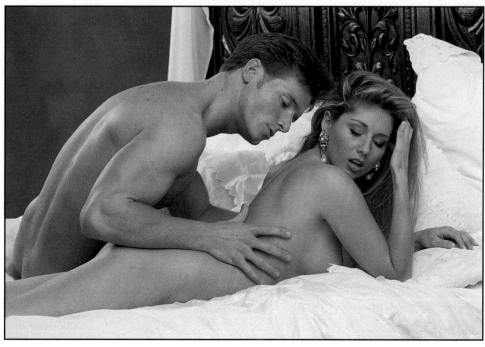

Some like the crisp freshness of white cotton sheets

with the lights out are shy—but it's possible they just can't stand the pain of a 100-watt spot bulb beaming in their eyes from above the bed. Soft, dim lighting is what most people appreciate in a romantic situation with their loved one. You can achieve it by putting low-watt bulbs in bedroom lamps; a dimmer switch which can lower the lights to twilight level; draping a large silk scarf over the shade of a bright light. Pink bulbs give lovers a rosy glow and candlelight gives naked bodies a golden aura that's sensuous and warm. But be careful not to put candles somewhere they might be blown over—for instance, on a window-sill—because of the fire risk. And make sure to blow them out before you go to sleep.

Bedroom temperatures are something to sort out between you—but it's no fun trying to be sexy when your teeth are chattering and your skin is bumpy and blue. If your mate insists on the windows being open when it's five-below-freezing outside, you

may insist on making love in flannel pyjamas, nightcap and bedsocks.

The feel of your surroundings can make the difference between a bedroom that adds to your sensual pleasure and one that is simply somewhere to sleep. So go for curtains, bedspread, carpets and furnishings that feel pleasurable to touch as well as looking inviting: velvets feel warm, luxurious and cosseting; satins and silks feel cool and slithery as bare skin; furry rugs are a treat for bare feet; mellow, polished wood invites you to run fingers over it. Exploring interesting surfaces with inquiring fingers increases your sensual skills, making you a more sensitive lover.

Delicious smells heighten desire, particularly if they are evocative of past romantic experience—like the smell of roses or jasmine below your window in a beautiful holiday spot. Or the fragrant whiff of pot pourri, incense or furniture polish, remembered from somewhere you once made unforgettable love. But even if you just freshen the air with a squirt or two of your favourite perfume or cologne it can make your love-nest more appealing.

But the bedroom is not the only location for love and one of the surest ways of spicing up a predictable sex life is to find new venues, even if they are only other rooms at home. The thrills of spontaneous sex can get lost once you settle into busy family life. But if you let yourselves get carried away every so often and end up finding ecstasy under the kitchen table or in the shower with your clothes on, it will put back the sparkle you once had. See if you can let sex happen wherever you are when the mood takes you.

Lovers like Melanie and Paul have become geniuses at creating new hotspots for passion around their small country cottage.

Melanie says: "The front door opens straight into the living room and is only a few steps away from our front gate. We were on our way to bed one night and were fooling around feeling frisky when we heard the neighbours chatting to some friends outside. We got behind the door and could hear every word as if they were in the room. That was when Paul started ripping my clothes off and really getting steamed up till we were naked, pressed against the door and there was no holding back.

"We were trying not to rattle the door or make a noise because the people outside were so close. It was just like doing it in the open when you're terrified someone will come past at the crucial moment—or in the living room of your parents' house when you hope they've gone to bed, but suddenly you hear them moving about. The fear definitely adds something—you're trying to hold back then suddenly you explode. It's amazing."

The swing on the porch outside their back door is another spot they've discovered for nookie that feels naughty. Paul says: "It's one of those swinging seats with a canopy and if you turn it round to face the house, there's no way anyone can see what you're up to. The first time we did it there, one Sunday after lunch, we were a bit tiddly and kept trying not to move too much in case we fell off. Now we've got the knack of doing it with Mel on my lap instead of trying to lie down, it works a treat."

The bathroom is one of the best settings for uninhibited passion at home because of all the opportunities it offers for lusty fun: bathing and showering together, lathering each other all over till you're frantic with desire, making love while warm water runs

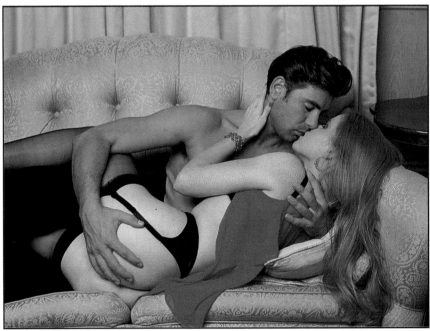

When we're having our early sexual experiences, a snog on the living room sofa is about as far as many of us get.

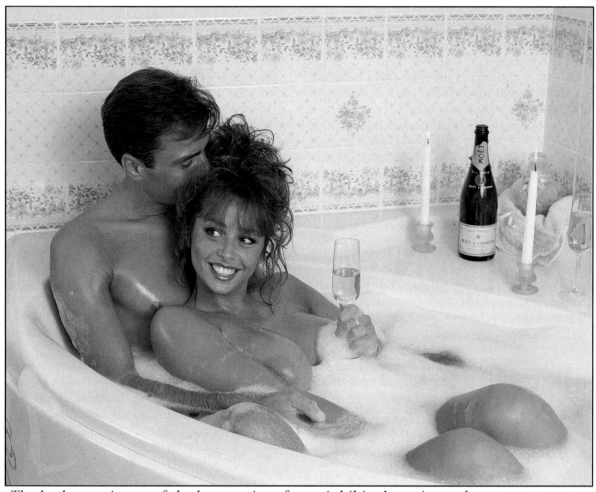

The bathroom is one of the best settings for uninhibited passion at home.

tantalisingly over your body, treating each other to a massage with body lotion. Not only that—you can lock the door without too many awkward questions from the kids.

Nancy and Tony have turned their suburban bathroom into an erotic haven where they can retreat for hours of pampered pleasure when the mood takes them. It was a small bedroom which they had converted with more than just bathing in mind. There's a king-size bath where both can fit in comfort, a luxurious shower with water jets coming from all sides, a big old sofa and acres of pale, deep-pile carpet. Besides the functional lighting, there are metal wall sconces which hold candles for more romantic moments.

"It's my favourite room. It feels a world away from the rest of the house. You can get in there and spend hours lounging round naked, even in winter, because it's so warm. Sometimes I just go in for a shower before bed but then Tony might come in with a nightcap and one thing leads to another. He's got magic fingers when it comes to massage. He'll offer to relax me with his top-to-toe special treatment and then, when I'm nearly asleep, I'll feel his lips and tongue take over and we're away. Other times he'll stretch out on a towel on the floor and I'll get to him with the body oil. Then we often end up in the shower, washing each other's hair, driving each other wild till we have to make love then and there."

Making long, luxurious love on a bearskin rug by a blazing log fire is a romantic fantasy shared by many. But when it comes to creating it in reality, couples often get put off by practical problems—they live in a modern house without a fireplace, an animal fur rug offends their wildlife-saving beliefs or they might be interrupted by the children.

If those are the kind of considerations stopping you, take heart from Rita and Ken's story of a night to remember. It was their wedding anniversary and they decided to celebrate at home on a wintry night by the glow of firelight. The lack of a fireplace was a problem they had to overcome.

"A two-bar radiator is not the same—but it's a start. The central heating kept the room warm so the radiator was just something glowing to add atmosphere. Then we turned off all the lights and filled the room with candles, some scented. Instead of a furry rug, we put the sofa cushions on the floor and threw a big soft blanket over them. We played our favourite classical guitar music, drank red wine and made love long and lazily into the night. It felt special and different—and that was the whole point," says Rita. "In fact, a real part of the pleasure was planning it beforehand. I felt quite keyed up, like I used to before an important date."

Outdoor loving has definite appeal to most people because of its close-to-nature feel. In one major national survey, two-thirds of the 7,000 who had taken part had made love in woods or fields. And what could be more perfect than feeling the sun caress your skin, watching puffs of cloud drift across an azure sky, breathing in the scent of new-mown hay—while sharing kisses with a loved one? The moment the sun comes out, so do lovers, filling parks, gardens, woods, fields and beaches with the sight of couples canoodling.

How can you get away with it? Incredibly easily—as long as you're discreet and not abandoning yourselves to unbridled passion in full view of passing crowds. Passers-by do look the other way and steer their children in other directions. Most people take a kindly view on the basis that they have either enjoyed similar frolics at some time, or would like to in future. You shouldn't get any hassle.

The main spoilers of al fresco romps are likely to be elements of nature like stinging insects, nettles, over-friendly cows, un-friendly farmers (specially if you leave their gates open or deposit your picnic rubbish in their hedges).

So head for secluded corners of parks and gardens and for fields free of grazing animals. Take a rug or groundsheet, cushions and insect-repellent.

If you're worried about prying eyes or the sudden arrival of others, wear clothes that keep you modest while allowing full and free lovemaking. A long skirt or dress that does up down the front can help disguise what's going on, so can outsize T-shirts, a beach towel or car rug.

"I've never forgotten making love on a beach in Cornwall," says housewife Rosemary. "It was late afternoon and all but deserted, just the odd person with a child or walking a dog. Clyde and I found a lovely spot where the sand was smooth and hard and we were between two large rocks which hid us almost entirely.

"We hadn't gone there with sex in mind, it just happened. We were enjoying the sound of the sea and the fresh, salty breeze in our hair, listening to the gulls squawking, a million miles from care. Suddenly we were wound round each other, I could feel him easing my shorts down in front, he was on top of me and we weren't going to stop ourselves. I had a quick glance towards some people in the distance but they were

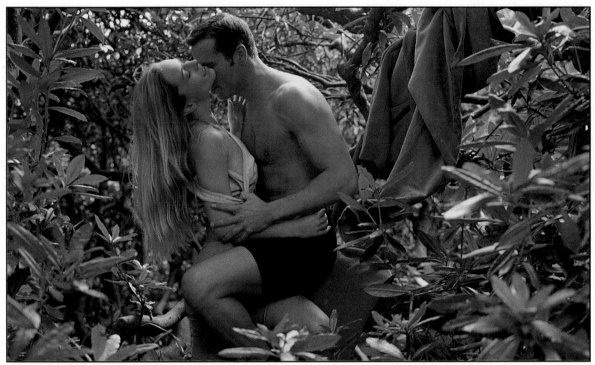

Outdoor loving has definite appeal to most people because of its close-to-nature feel.

playing with their dog—and anyway, I was beyond worrying, out of control, ecstatic.

"When it was over, we just lay where we were, dazed and dreamy, aware of the sun setting and the day getting cool. There was no one around and I said to Clyde, 'I want to remember this moment forever.'"

Sex on the sand has only one drawback—the sand itself, if it gets into the more intimate parts of your body. It's worth making sure you have a towel, a sunbed or even a li-lo to lie on so you won't get scratched to pieces—or have sand falling out of your knickers for days afterwards.

For 30-year-old electrician Gary, the most adventurous sex he ever had was in the sea. "It felt incredible as the water lapped round, she floated on her back and I could hold her in my arms, completely weightless. I noticed her nipples were hard as she put her arms round my neck and wrapped her legs around me. We were out in the deep with no one near so it was easy to slip out of our swimming gear. We floated together, her on top, feeling each other get more and more worked up. It was an amazing feeling of freedom—there were masses of people on the beach but they were too far away to see what we were up to.

"When we came, it was magic. It felt as if we were exploding with pleasure, gasping and spluttering and laughing all at once."

Picnics are perfect for long, lazy afternoons of love, as long as you can find somewhere you won't be disturbed. Your own back garden can be best of all, as long as there's a shady tree, secluded corner or high fence to protect you from nosy neighbours.

Finger food like strawberries, grapes, cherries, cheese nibbles, nuts, is sexiest for popping into each other's mouth or serving from intimate parts of your body. Keep wine or fruit juice in a bucket of ice—you can always use an ice cube to make your lover's nipples tingle or to freshen up their naughty bits.

Make a daisy chain and thread it round your lover's secret places or tickle them to ecstasy with a long frond of grass or haystalk. Make barnyard noises as you get in the mood to behave like animals.

If it's a sweltering day or if you are on holiday somewhere hot, don't forget your suntan lotion—applying it to each other's tenderest parts can make for sizzling sex play. And beware of falling asleep in the sun afterwards. The sunburn that may result will make your skin sting, so that loving becomes just too painful.

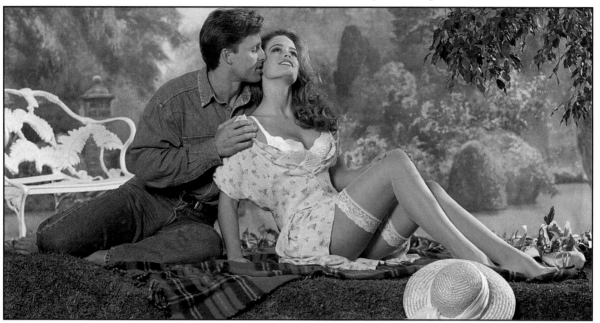

Picnics are perfect for long, lazy afternoons of love.

The danger of discovery makes many lovers shiver with delight at indulging in sex in public places. When sex feels forbidden, it's irresistible; that is why so many randy couples get carried away by the thrill of risking being caught in the act.

Why else would you want to make love in an aeroplane loo and join the infamous Mile High Club? It is extremely uncomfortable and enrages other passengers queueing with their legs crossed outside.

These love locations that will either make you wince or grab your mate have been claimed by men and women in surveys:

The lift at work
In a restaurant loo
In a phone box
A station waiting room
A bowling green
A cave
A pub floor
On a roller-coaster
On a window ledge
On an historic monument

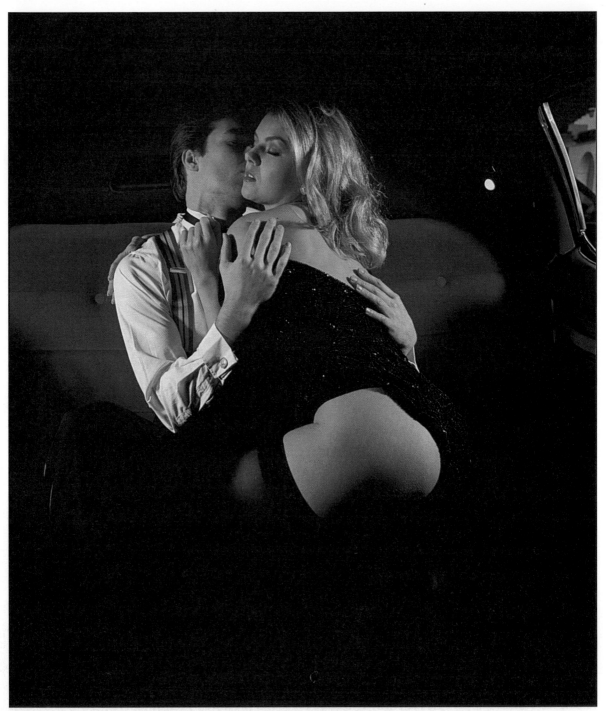

Cars that score at the mating game are those with big back seats, soft upholstery, good springs and enough space to manoeuvre without getting caught up in gearsticks, steering wheels and foot pedals.

CARS: A SUPERSEX ROAD TEST

After the bedroom and the living room, cars are the most popular love-spot. Research has found that just over seven out of ten of us have made love in a car at least once. This is probably because young lovers often have nowhere more private to go.

Cars that score at the mating game are those with big back seats, soft upholstery, good springs and enough space to manoeuvre without getting caught up in gearsticks, steering wheels and foot pedals.

Top points for passion include:

Astra Max: The speedy van that always passes you on the motorway has obvious appeal to fast types who keep a mattress in the back and install curtains for privacy. Popular with plumbers and surfers.

American and British classic cars of the 50s and 60s with bench front seats—about the only vehicles suitable for front-seat sex.

Fiat Punto and most of today's small hatchbacks where the back seat flattens, making room to lie down.

Saab Turbo: Fold the back seats down and there is rear space more than six feet long. Great for a tumble with someone tall.

Range Rover: With its high roof, comfy seats and good springs, it's almost as good as your living room sofa.

Rolls Royce, Bentley, Mercedes S class: Luxury loving on wheels—but if you've got one of these, you've probably got a mansion full of bedrooms at your disposal.

Motors mostly suitable for midgets or contortionists:

Porsche, Mazda RX7: Virtually no back seat and severe danger of injury if you try to do it in the confined space up front.

McLaren F1: the world's most expensive car is a three-seater with the driver in the middle and you have to be double-jointed to get in or out of it, let alone try anything more gymnastic than holding hands or kissing.

Robin Reliant: the problem with a three-wheeler is that if you rock it too vigorously, it might fall over.

Rocket: Sporty, flash and very fast—but its two seats are one behind the other which rules out most hanky-panky entirely.

Or you could just stick to taxis, like bank clerk Chris and his girlfriend Sue, who found that taxi drivers tend to turn a blind eye when lovers get to grips with each other on the back seat.

Chris says: "You can keep respectable in your coats and jackets while you rip off each other's undies out of sight of the rear-vision mirror."

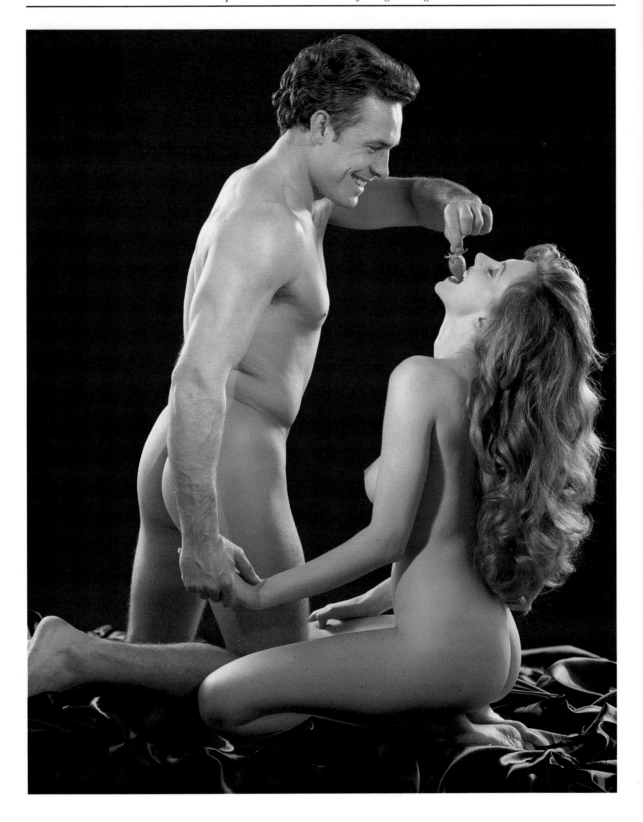

SEX DRIVE
The Owner's Manual

Sex drive is the unseen power which motivates us all, ticking over till it explodes into ecstasy. And it takes only the smallest sensual trigger—a look, a touch, a sound, a smell—to fire up feelings of lust and longing.

From that first switch-on, we are driven towards the pinnacle of passion we hope to reach with our chosen lover.

But some of us turn on to those loving feelings far more frequently and strongly than others. Just as we have different appetites for food, different energies for physical activity, so we all have different levels of arousal

In the early stages of a love affair, lust-levels are usually at their peak on both sides. We can't keep our hands off each other, every touch sending us into sexual overdrive as we race on to an explosive climax.

Some lusty lovers never lose that feeling. But many others find their sex drive slackening as relationships slide into routines where they make love out of habit rather than desire.

Pressures of everyday life—problems at work, family hassles, money—are also passion-killers.

But if your sex drive is sputtering, there is plenty you can do to revive it. To start, you can rev up your raunch-rating by tuning into your own and your mate's innermost needs and desires.

• Think about the most exhilarating, heart-pounding, skin-tingling turn-ons you have ever experienced. Like the time you got carried away caressing each other intimately with your bare toes under a cafe table, and had to finish by making love on the floor. Remembering what it was that gave you such sexual ecstasy should stir you to achieve it again.

• Tell *him* if you dream of being overpowered, roughly stripped and threatened with punishment—before being loved till it hurts. It should bring out the beast in your man.

• Tell *her* if you'd like to lay her out on a pile of silk cushions and slather her in perfumed lotions, like Cleopatra being made ready for a night of love with Antony. You'd like to tickle her with feathers, tantalise her with your tongue and tease her till she cries out for you to ravish her.

• If one of you is ever-ready for sex and the other takes a long, slow warm-up before starting to sizzle, practise pacing yourselves. One can hold back while gently rousing the other with kisses and cuddles.

• A glass of wine and a sexy video can relax and put you in the mood—especially if you watch while lying naked on a sofa or on a furry rug by a fire.

• Go even further—be the stars of your own blue movie by videoing your bedtime gymnastics. Or take polaroid pictures of each other in raunchy poses.

• Romance your mate with little loving gestures to show you care—at any and every moment of the day, not just bedtime.

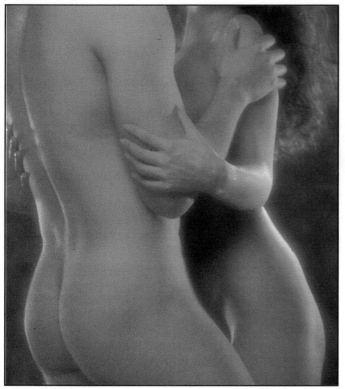

Touching almost any part of your lover's skin can be an erotic experience.

Put your hand in his pocket and squeeze his loose change. Stroke her bottom, exploring every curve. It will make you feel permanently warm towards each other—a way of keeping both your sexual motors purring perfectly.

Now turn on to the sexquisite pleasures of the senses:

Start by thinking about sex when you're on your own—what you long to do to your partner, what you ache for them to do to you. It will put you in the mood, and stir you into action. Find out, by talking intimately together, what are the touches, sights, sounds, tastes and smells that turn you both on. Then stir your senses with the following sensual guide.

TOUCH

The skin is the body's sexiest organ after the brain. It stretches over more than two square metres and is alive with nerve endings. So touching almost any part of your lover's skin can be an erotic experience.

Here are 10 Tantalising Touches to Turn You On.

1. Stroke your naked lover with a piece of long grass—down the insides of their arms, up the insides of the legs. Round their nipples, over their stomach and down to more intimate parts. It will drive them to a writhing frenzy, ready to lock bodies for an ecstatic finish.

2. Give your mate an all-over massage with scented oil, keeping away from their obvious erogenous zones at first. Make sure the room is very warm and work your way lovingly round their body till they're totally relaxed and aching for your fingers to reach sexier parts.

3. Kiss, lick and nuzzle their face, neck and ears till it makes them delirious with pleasure. Trace little nibbling kisses over forehead, temples, eyelids and round the outside of the lips. Gently suck the ear-lobes, breathe lightly into the ears and nuzzle the back of the neck.

4. Stroke and caress each other while fully dressed. It rubs you up the right way if you're wearing something silky which slips seductively over the skin's surface. Now slide your hands inside each other's clothes and fiddle with the naughtiest bits you can reach.

5. Share a lingering shower. Soap each other all over, exploring every nook and cranny. Wash each other's hair till it's squeaky clean. Then, when you're both hot and slippery, wrap yourselves round each other and make love as the water splashes over you.

6. Your hands and feet are more supersensitive than you think. Sucking your lov-

er's fingers and toes can bring them such ecstasy they'll be begging you to stop and grind your bodies together in a loving frenzy.

7. Playful pinching, tweaking, slapping and squeezing adds the spice of pain to the pleasure of lovemaking. It can stimulate desire by making the blood rush to the skin's surface and heightening excitement. Lots of women like their nipples squeezed quite hard, and men their buttocks grabbed till they hurt, in the final thrusts of passion.

8. For her: use your whole body, specially your nipples, lips, hair and inside thighs to stroke and caress every inch of his naked body.

9. For him: pretend to eat her alive by nibbling and nipping her all over, especially breasts, buttocks and naughty bits, till she throbs with longing.

10. Use your tongue to lick your lover all over, giving little flicking licks and long strokes that are wet and tender. Caress every part you can reach, probing deeply wherever you can. Get them to do the same for you, till you're both aching to go further.

SIGHT

Men more than women are sexually stirred by the sights around them, seeing come-ons in every glance, every peep of stocking top or lacy bra. Women who've worked this out can send their man sexstatic by letting him feast his eyes on what's to come.

So treat him to any, some or all of the following eyefuls:

1. Sit beside him so he can see from the way your blouse falls open that you're not wearing a bra.

2. When you cross and uncross your legs, let him see a stretch of suspender—and a flash of no-knickers.

3. Walk round at home wearing nothing but a T-shirt that barely covers your bum.

4. Make sure he's watching when you fondle your naked breasts in the bathroom mirror.

5. Greet him at the door wearing nothing but a towel—and drop it as soon as the door's shut. Bend over very slowly to pick it up, then let it trail on the floor as you walk ahead of him.

6. Take his eyes off the telly by stripping seductively in the living room. Unbutton your top slowly and slide it off your shoulders, then wiggle out of your skirt so you're left in your sauciest basque, suspenders, stockings and highest heels. Take each piece off very slowly, perching on his knee to remove your stockings—or let him do it for you.

7. Do the hoovering in the nude.

8. Cook the evening meal wearing nothing but a bare top, a frilly apron and high heels.

9. Wear a silky shirt when it's cold so you're covered up—but your erect nipples will be a welcome sight to your man.

10. Meet him for a drink wearing nothing under your coat—and surprise him by letting him help you out of it back home.

SOUND

Sexy sounds send shivers down your spine, whether they come from throbbing music or the sound of waves crashing on a deserted shore.

You'll know the music that turns your mate into a sex maniac, whether it's Ravel's *Bolero,* Madonna or Meatloaf. But there are other sounds that can have you tearing at each other's clothes.

1. Try phoning your lover at work and describing in detail the sex act you long to perform with them—say you want to tie them to the bed with silk scarves then kiss them lovingly all over.

2. Or whisper rude suggestions in their ear as you're shopping in the supermarket— talk dirty in your softest, breathiest voice about what you might do with a banana, a mango or a Mars bar.

3. Play jungle sounds on the bedroom stereo to hot up the atmosphere—and make your mate want to rip off your loin-cloth and

follow their animal instincts.

4. Try the tinkle of wind-chimes if your mate likes to imagine a breath of fresh air on their bare bits—while playing Tarzan and Jane on the living room carpet.

TASTE

Set your lover's taste buds tingling by popping saucy titbits in their mouth—your tongue, for instance. (But before any mouth-to-mouth activity, make sure your teeth are clean and your breath sweet.)

1. Give your mate a taste treat by feeding them strawberries from your mouth to theirs.

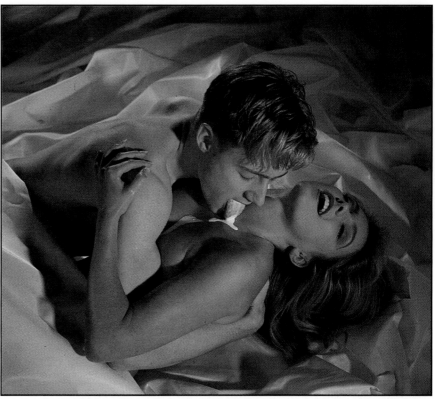

Put whipped cream on any part of your body that likes to be licked—and let your partner's tongue do the trick.

2. Share a chocolate bar by putting an end in each of your mouths and working towards the middle. Then make a meal of licking melted chocolate off each other's lips.

3. Trickle chocolate sauce over your mate's nipples and down to their tenderer parts. Then tenderly lick it off.

4. Put whipped cream on any part of your body that likes to be licked—and let your partner's tongue do the trick.

5. The sexiest way to sip after-dinner liqueurs is from your lover's lips. Take turns to take a mouthful of your favourite tipple, kiss and let it run into your partner's mouth.

6. Tease each other by eating a feast of rude food—anything succulent that looks like male and female sexy bits. Eat it in the same lusty style you'd devour the real thing. Then move on to the real thing.

SMELL

The familiar scent of the one you love, whether it's their natural, just-bathed fragrance, their favourite after-shave or perfume, can fire you with animal lust. So can scents which have filled the air at memorable moments of passion—the heady smell of incense, scented candles or night-scented flowers you've breathed while locked in uninhibited lovemaking.

1. Squirt your usual scent on a pair of your knickers or boxer shorts and slip them in your partner's pocket.

2. Sense your lover all around as you drive to work—by spraying their perfume or after-shave in your car.

3. Choose a scent that turns you both on and always use candles, room spray, scented oil or incense in that fragrance in the bedroom.

4. Wear a sweater or shirt your lover has just worn. You'll be sniffing their sexy scent all day.

5. Spray your own regular cologne or perfume on the cuffs of your lover's shirt—every time they raise a hand, they'll turn on to your smell.

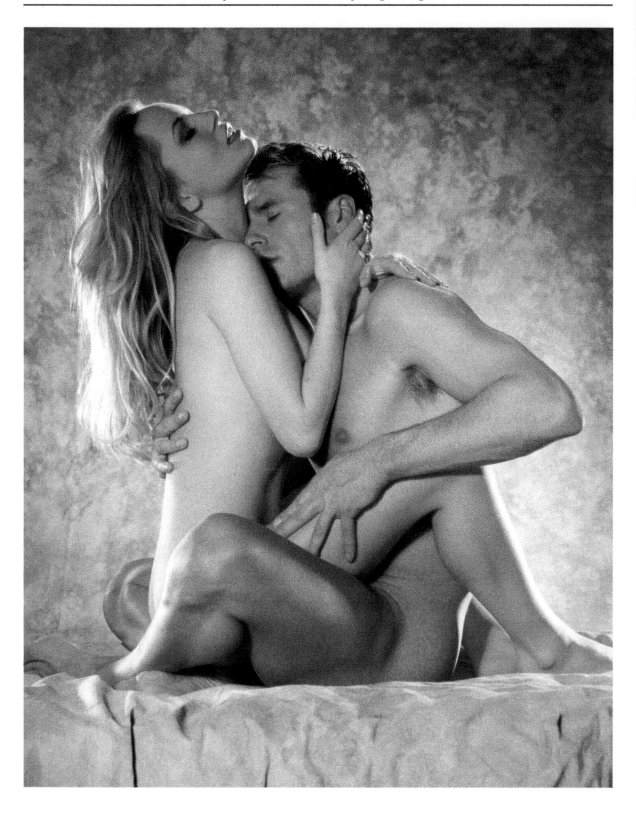

THE BIG O
Orgasm, or making the earth move

Fire-rockets scudding across the heavens. Volcanoes shooting their contents skywards. The earth shuddering and lurching beneath you. Trains hurtling into tunnels and waterfalls crashing on rocks. Stupendous, spectacular, describe it how you will, that's an orgasm for you—if you get the general drift. But reading about it can only ever give you the vaguest idea of what it feels like to actually have an orgasm.

The French call it *'petit mort'* meaning 'little death', presumably because for those brief moments of utter ecstasy one definitely feels out of this world.

Birth-control campaigner Marie Stopes, whose book *Married Love* was a shocker in the Twenties when it promoted the pleasures of sex for women, described it this way: "The half-swooning sense of flux which overtakes the spirit in that eternal moment at the apex of rapture." But this is decidedly dodgy stuff—she wrote it while still a virgin.

What you can be fairly sure of is that you'll enjoy that mysterious sensation which can be anything from a dizzying, out-of-control body seizure to an all-over shiver of excitement, concentrated enough to make your toes curl. It's a different feeling for each of us and we all enjoy different kinds of orgasm at different times, from the prolonged, roller-coaster version to the three-second, whizz-bang-it's-over job.

It is also perfectly possible to make love without reaching orgasm and still have a good time. Instead of finishing with an explosive climax, snuggling up to sleep in the arms of someone who loves you is a happy ending that's hard to beat. On the other hand, thrashing away trying to achieve orgasm for one or both of you can be a hell of a disappointing experience if either someone isn't in the mood or can't maintain their enthusiasm.

Not that long ago, women were presumed to be the sex that didn't need a blow-your-head-off climax to their lovemaking. Mostly they lay back and took what came to them. Victorian women supposedly thought of England while their men enjoyed their conjugal rights. Up until the Sixties, women frequently faked their orgasms while thinking shopping lists and how not to get pregnant. Then came the Pill and womens' rights and suddenly the only thing on womens' minds was how to have an orgasm or, preferably, how to have lots of them—the multiple orgasm being the ultimate pleasure goal.

Men, used to achieving their own sexual satisfaction in the vague hope that what was good for them was at least okay for women, now found they *really* had to perform. Give her an orgasm or else. Give her more than one and you're Superlover. Women, having discovered the possibility of the orgasm, have been insisting on it ever since. It is now reckoned that 95 per cent of women can have orgasms—and a hot-blooded 75 per cent of them can have multiples. Which means a lot of men are having to work their socks off in bed to give women the satisfaction they demand.

Nothing unfair about that, you might think. After all, men had sexual pleasure to themselves till quite recently. But it's the revelation by scientists that women can have so many more orgasms than men that has freaked the fellas. In tests carried out by Drs William Hartman and Marilyn Fithian at the Centre for Marital and Sexual Studies, Long Beach, California, the female

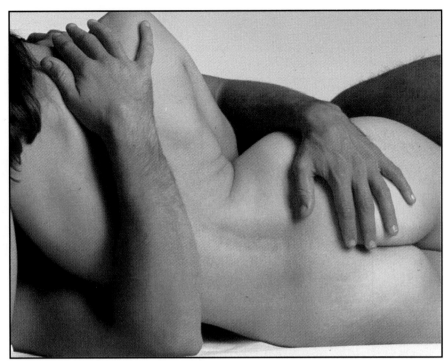

The sexual organs and timing may be different in men and women but both bodies react in more or less the same way.

record for orgasms in one hour was a gasp-making 134 while the male record was a mere (or magnificent, looking at it from another angle) 16.

Just as it was not thought possible for women to enjoy sex as much as men, it was also thought impossible for men to have multiple orgasms. But Drs Hartman and Fithian insist that they can. Not just lusty young studs who can get roused without much effort after brief pauses between climaxes but men who can thrill to orgasms over and over before finally letting go and ejaculating.

So now we all know—men CAN hold back to give not only their partners but themselves maximum pleasure. But they mostly have to work at it, quite hard, because biologically they are geared to reach their climax at more than twice the speed of women. Men reach their point of no return in an average eleven minutes while it's es-

timated that a woman takes an average 27 minutes to reach a climax.

NOW FOR THE TECHNICAL DETAILS.

The sexual organs and timing may be different in men and women but both bodies react in more or less the same way when it's all-systems-go towards orgasm.

What happens to *her* is this:

1. Her vagina starts to get very juicy as moisture gathers on its walls and also seeps from glands near its entrance. At the same time, her labia start to part and swell, getting ready for the penis to enter.

2. Her pulse starts to race and blood pressure rises.

3. A pinkish flush starts to glow on her stomach and breasts.

4. As her whole system steams up, she begins to breathe as if she's just sprinted for a bus.

5. Her clitoris pops up, doubling in size, in a mini-version of what the penis does.

6. Her inner labia go red or even as dark as burgundy.

7. Her nipples grow hard and erect and the pink circle around them, the areola, flushes with a deeper colour.

8. Her face usually twists into an expression of pain as if her partner is standing on her foot and she's too agonised to tell him.

9. Her brain goes into switch-off mode as she lets go control of her body.

10. Her arms and legs go into spasm-mode as her pelvis pushes rhythmically against his.

11. She may let out a blood-curdling scream, enough to wake the neighbours.

12. Her toes may spread or curl up.

13. The muscles round her bottom may get the flutters.

14. From the moment she's ready for it to the moment of climax can take anything from 15 seconds to about four minutes.

What happens to *him* is as follows:

1. His penis becomes erect due to a concentration of blood which pours into it and becomes trapped, forcing it to stiffen and lengthen to its full extent. It also darkens to a purplish colour.

2. His heart and pulse rates go zooming up.

3. His breathing gets heavier.

4. His body, like a woman's, may get a rosy glow on the skin due to the speeding up of pulse and heart rates.

5. His nipples will harden.

6. His testicles will swell noticeably and the scrotum will contract so they no longer hang down but are held right up near the base of the penis.

7. His face muscles will tighten into a look of severe strain as if he's trying to lift a steel girder single-handed.

8. His bottom will clench tightly and his back and thighs will momentarily seize up.

9. His toes, like hers, may fan out and curl up.

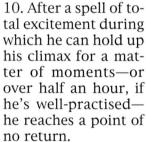

10. After a spell of total excitement during which he can hold up his climax for a matter of moments—or over half an hour, if he's well-practised— he reaches a point of no return.

11. The semen finds its way to the base of the penis, ready for ejaculation.

12. The urethra and prostate gland contract strongly to send the semen shooting out of the penis in several quick bursts. And it's all over for him.

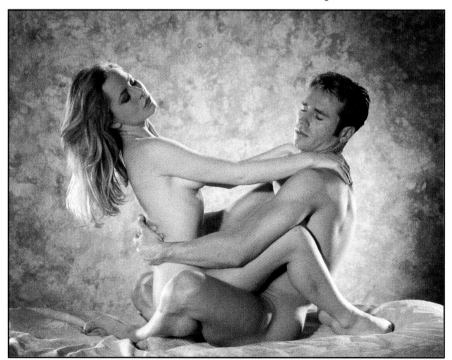

His body, like a woman's, may get a rosy glow on the skin due to the speeding up of pulse and heart rates.

BE A SUPERLOVER

Like the size of a man's equipment, the bedtime stamina of either partner is unimportant compared with their loving feelings, their caring give-and-take, their desire for each other's pleasure and happiness.

But there are love-workouts both sexes can do to help produce gold-medal performances between the sheets. We're talking supersex here, which can be sublime for both—providing it doesn't turn into competitive sport. So don't count your orgasms, enjoy the quality of them.

It's all to do with muscle-power in the pelvic area of both men and women. Exercises originally devised in the Fifties to help women's bodies tighten up after childbirth have been found to have an amazing effect on men's ability to control ejaculation, helping them to hold fire almost as long as they want or as long as it takes to bring their partner to orgasm.

Easy to do, the exercises are often called 'Kegels' after Dr Arnold Kegel who prescribed them for his women patients. Any woman who has had a baby will know the ones—you clench and unclench the muscles you use when you're trying to hold back from peeing. The idea is to get the vagina back to its original shape. But it has been found to do far more for a woman's love life than that.

Enthusiastic Kegel-practitioners were overjoyed when they discovered some unexpected side-effects: they were able to reach orgasm more easily and to peak over and over in an ecstatic series of climaxes. Some even discovered an ancient Eastern skill, used by women described as kabbazah, who could bring a man to ecstasy simply by taking his penis into her vagina and flexing these muscles—while he lay back and did nothing. Not a bump, not a grind. (She also shared the ecstatic experience, it should be added hastily).

But then, the mind-blowing news for men. They too could get Kegel-power. By doing the same clenching of the (let's get technical) pubococcygeous muscle—it stretches from the pubic bone to the base of the spine—they could build up the skill to delay ejaculation while thrilling to a series of multiple orgasms. And just in case you thought that was progress, apparently the Chinese have been onto this trick for about 5,000 years and it is also well-established in the repertoire of Indian and Middle-Eastern lovers.

With the Chinese, stopping their semen escaping was considered as vital as not losing blood. They thought of it as a life force that needed to be stored, not spent.

Sex-watchers Hartman and Fithian say most men can train themselves to be multi-orgasmic—and 12 per cent already are, either by training or lucky chance. The Californian doctors base this on tests on 282 men whose bodily reactions during orgasm they measured using a dynograph, a gadget that can measure all the body's flutterings and surges.

Now Hartman claims he can teach any man to orgasm in multiples. Here's how:

• The secret is to clench the pelvic muscles tight for 15 seconds when ejaculation is near. And the muscle control a man needs for this can be got from doing his daily Kegels.

• Start with 20-a-day as follows: for the first ten, clench for three-seconds each, relax and clench again. Then do ten quick ones, clench-unclench-clench and so on, without pausing in between.

• Just like building muscle-power in the gym, once that's easy, add another set of 20-a-day.

• The best thing about these exercises is that you can do them anywhere: at your desk, in a traffic jam, on the bus, while watching telly.

• Build up gradually till you can do 200 a day in sets of 20—and your reward should exceed your wildest sexpectations.

Women prepared to work on their Kegels may fancy the idea of what is said to be the ultimate sex thrill—doing it the kabbazah way. That means using the muscles around the vagina to grip the penis, squeeze and release, without moving any other part of the body.

• Choose a position with deep penetration so you don't have to wriggle and push for maximum contact.

• He mustn't move a muscle but lie or sit very still just feeling the sexy sensations of her internal muscles.

• Stillness from both partners is a must.

• As she contracts and lets go those well-primed pelvic muscles he will start to throb with excitement.

• His throbbing will excite her more and more, so both may reach a state of unbearable excitement after about 15 minutes.

• This should be followed by a peaceful, glowing, very alive state

• She gets those magic muscles working again and after about another 15 minutes, it's said to be an orgasm like no other.

AND AFTER ALL THAT, WHAT?

A woman's body, slower than a man's to reach peak excitement, also takes longer to go back to normal.

Once the wild thrashing around has stopped, she lies back in a warm glow of satisfaction and exhaustion as all her muscles lose their tension and her breathing slows to a relaxed rate.

Gradually, the mottled flush on the front of her body fades as the rush of blood to the surface subsides. Her breasts, clitoris and labia all lose their rosy colour and sexy swelling. Her vagina stops tingling and she may feel a little glum and in need of cuddles and reassurance.

It takes about six minutes for her to wind down in this way.

A man starts to get that shrinking feeling as soon as he has spurted out the final burst of semen. The blood starts departing from the penis, which begins to soften, and the testicles drop back to their original position dangling behind the penis. This only takes about a minute.

At this stage, a man often feels rather dejected, drained, and in need of a good sleep to help his recovery. He can't rise to the occasion for some time and his sexual equipment needs a Do Not Touch sign due to its tender state.

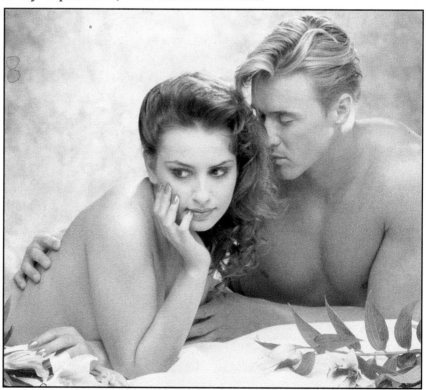

All her muscles lose their tension and her breathing slows to a relaxed rate.

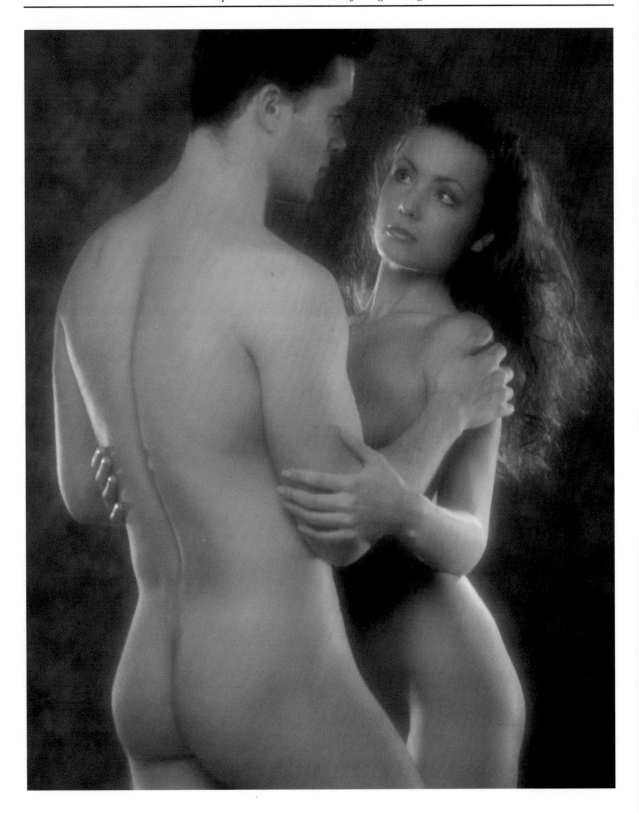

THE BIG OH-NO!

Your mate wants something and you don't

Whatever consenting adults do to give each other bedtime pleasure is okay—as long as no one's doing anything they don't want to do. That is the gospel according to the sexperts.

It sounds clear cut but when it comes to the crunch there is going to be a lot of sliding round the issue. Who's asking and who's giving a definite yes or no? It doesn't work like that at all.

One of you may have a secret desire to be, say, tied down with silken bonds then tantalised to near-orgasm by a partner's stroking and tweaking. Nothing sinister or perverse, just a playful game to add a frisson of naughtiness to an otherwise routine sex life. But how do you tell your mate? Try to put that matter-of-factly over the steak-and-chips. No, what you'll do is fantasise about it, long for it, hint that you'd like to try it, hope it will somehow cross your lover's mind. You might even show a video with titillating bondage scenes or start one of those conversations that begins, "I wonder what people get out of tying each other up, don't you?"

At which point you may get one of those warning looks from your mate and a very frosty, "No, I don't ever wonder." And you know your chances of putting this new kick into bedtime frolics are minus zero.

And then, suppose it's you being asked, wheedled or seduced into fulfilling some sexual need of your mate's that you don't happen to fancy. Or you don't think you'd fancy and you're not rushing to find out. Oh no, you groan inwardly, not *that!*

Depending on how comfortably intimate you are, you may be able to talk through each other's sexual tastes and distastes and decide what each of you is prepared to do for the other and what is totally taboo. Or, more likely, you will do your best to avoid all mention of the sexual practice you don't like the sound of in the hope that you won't ever be asked about it again. It will then become a no-go area between you so that one will feel deprived of what they believe is a pleasurable sex act; the other will feel dread at the possibility of it coming up for discussion.

But a problem you cannot talk about will rarely go away. It's more likely to fester and break out in ways that could poison your relationship.

So, for your future happiness as a couple, it would be better to find a way of coping with the Big Oh-No! between you, whether it's something as basic as one of you not wanting to undress in front of the other, a distaste for oral sex or something more likely to cause fear and doubt, like bondage, spanking or threesomes.

ORAL SEX

Nicky, a 30-year-old teacher, had never thought much about oral sex and never tried it till after she'd been married a couple of years. "Ben didn't say anything but every now and then he would somehow manoeuvre into position kneeling over my head with his penis waving in my face. I found it quite alarming and claustrophobic and wanted to push him away. But I didn't want to hurt his feelings so I'd kiss it as quickly as I could and hold it for a bit. But there was no way I was going to put it in my mouth.

"He could tell I wasn't keen but he

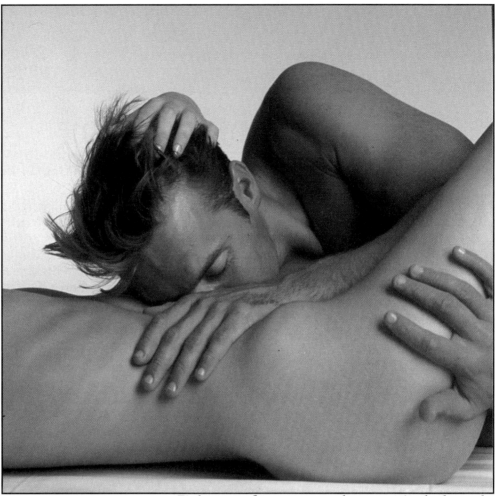

Eight out of ten men and women include oral sex as a regular part of lovemaking.

didn't try to talk about it and I didn't want to ask him. He gave up trying for a bit but then he started trying the other way round, licking and nibbling me. At first I found it ticklish and irritating and would have to push him off after a bit. But then either he got better at it or I got used to it—I would lie there hoping he could keep it up forever. It felt *so* amazing.

"That was when I thought, what the hell, he's doing this for me, I'd better try to do him the same favour. I waited till he was lying propped up on his side so I could do it without being under him and I found it

wasn't so bad at all. Specially when I could look up and see his face and he was smiling like an angel—it hit me how much happiness I was giving him and somehow my hesitation disappeared. I haven't got to the stage where I'd let him come in my mouth. I still don't fancy that but I might pluck up courage one day."

If it's you who longs to be treated to oral sex (a very common Big Oh-No!) it's not an unreasonable request to make of your mate. Both fellatio (when the man is the receiver) and cunnilingus (the woman gets the favour) are generally agreed to be gourmet dishes on the sex menu, either as the entree that makes you ravenous for the main course or as the main course. Both men and women are brought to shimmering peaks of satisfaction by oral sex, possibly because you can treat each other separately and therefore give 100 per cent attention to your partner's orgasm. What could be a more loving and generous gesture?

But lots of people feel funny about it, probably women more so than men. When asked in sex surveys what thrills they would like to enjoy more often, men always put in a mass bid for more blow-jobs (as fellatio is commonly known). Which does indicate that women are often reluctant to open their mouths to their man's pride and joy.

There are also people of both sexes who are either prepared to give but not receive oral sex—or the other way around. It seems that some men are worried a woman could get nasty and sink her teeth in. And some women fear that the taste and smell of their love organs would be uninviting.

But the first fear is only rational if a man is making love to a woman with sadistic tendencies. And the second is unfounded as long as a woman washes regularly—the taste of her love juices is said to be pleasantly unusual.

In more timid times, oral sex was certainly thought by some to be kinky and unhealthy. But now we know it's a very normal pastime. However, if you feel finicky or in any way freaked by it, that's not going to help. And, worst of all, if you have been forced into it by a selfish or insensitive lover, that could be most off-putting of all.

Then again, if you love somebody truly, madly, deeply, you want to do everything possible to make them happy. So you have to ask yourself if you might overcome your inhibition and try what eight out of ten men and women do as a regular part of love-making.

Use a position that is comfortable and unthreatening—having someone crawl over your face in order to get their love machinery within reach of your mouth is as off-putting as having a hamburger stuffed in your mouth if you're a vegetarian. Let the receiver lie down and the giver kneel by their side. Or the receiver can sit in a chair while the giver kneels on the floor in front of them.

Little by little is a good way of going about it. Start with gentle kissing of your partner's most intimate parts.

A woman should use her hands as well—imagining she's holding an ice-cream cone and savouring every lick of her tongue over and around the tip is one way of explaining how to do it.

When she's ready to take her man's most precious possession into her mouth she should keep her teeth well out of the way.

A couple should agree beforehand on whether or not she wants him to ejaculate in her mouth. What she should know is: it won't drown her as it's only a teaspoonful; it tastes rather salty but not offensive; it is completely harmless to swallow; it has very few calories.

He should warn her when he's about to come.

If he is treating her, he should also keep his teeth clear of her delicate sex organs. Kissing and licking are more sensuous than sucking. Inserting his tongue in her vagina can be highly erotic for both.

Simultaneous oral sex, known as '69', can be sublime but is not recommended for beginners as there is so much going on it can be confusing. Being driven wild at one end while trying to keep your mind on the job you're doing at the other is better tried once you're both well-practised at performing this sex act individually.

HEALTH WARNINGS: Never blow down a penis, it can cause infection. Don't put your mouth near your mate's sex organs if you have any kind of mouth infection—or they have any kind of genital infection.

BONDAGE

For Helen, the thought of being tied by her wrists and ankles to her bedposts, leaving her spread-eagled and helpless in husband Tom's power, was a fantasy she often enjoyed during their love sessions. She would grasp the bedhead and writhe under his touch, as if she was already shackled. "I thought that was probably as far as it would ever go since I felt it was too kinky to ask Tom. But then we saw a movie where this woman was tied up while her lover did everything you could imagine to excite her. I was so turned on by it my body was literally aching while I watched. Tom suddenly turned to me and said, 'I think you'd like that, wouldn't you?' I suppose he noticed I was breathing heavily or something.

"When it was over, he led me to the bedroom and asked if I had four silk scarves. I knew straight away what was coming. I couldn't wait. I let him undress me down to my knickers and lead me to the bed where he tied me firmly to the posts. At first he lay on top of me in his clothes, rubbing himself against me and telling me what he was going to do to me, in great detail.

"Then he got up and started undressing, never taking his eyes off me. He walked over and ran his fingers ever so lightly over my nipples then let his fingertips trail, hardly touching, round my breasts and down my stomach, very slowly. He did it for ages, just going down to the top of my pants. Then he started stroking my thighs and easing his fingers into my knickers. I was wriggling and writhing all over the place and longing for him to just take me.

"Suddenly he grabbed my knickers and ripped them sideways, tearing them off me. By now I was throbbing and begging him, 'Now, NOW...Please!'

"Once he was inside me I just exploded. I was like a grenade going off. It was the best sex I'd ever had.

"We do it every now and then and it's still electrifying for me. I think it's because Tom's such a gentle person that it's such a turn-on to suddenly feel he's taking me by force."

Bondage is harmless as long as both partners find it fun and no one gets hurt. It is a way of making dreams come true for many women who are turned on by the thought of swashbuckling heroes having their wicked way with them. And just as many men are tickled by being tied up and tantalised.

For some, it is a way of letting themselves enjoy sex without guilt—if they're having things done to them which they can't prevent, they are not responsible.

As long as you are with a trusted partner whom you know will stop if you want them to, it is a safe sex game. Just remember:

Never tie anyone too tightly or with rough rope or wire or anything that might hurt. Use knots you can undo easily.

Agree on a code-word that means you are serious when you want to stop—and you're not just yelling for them to stop as part of reaching a climax too soon

SEX TOYS

Finding a vibrator on his girlfriend's bedside table was a shock for transport worker, Steve, 26, who feared he'd failed her as a lover: "She never seemed to have any trouble coming and she was always saying I was fantastic in bed, so what was I meant to think? That she was giving herself a top up when I wasn't around? When I asked her about it, she looked guilty as if I wasn't meant to find out. How could she do it with that thing when she had a man in the house? When I said that to her, she didn't know what to say and we had a big row."

Vibrators are popular sex toys which give a buzz to a lot of women's sex lives—and consequently can add to their men's pleasure as well. They are mostly penis-shaped, battery-operated and can be slid into the vagina or laid on the clitoris or used on the

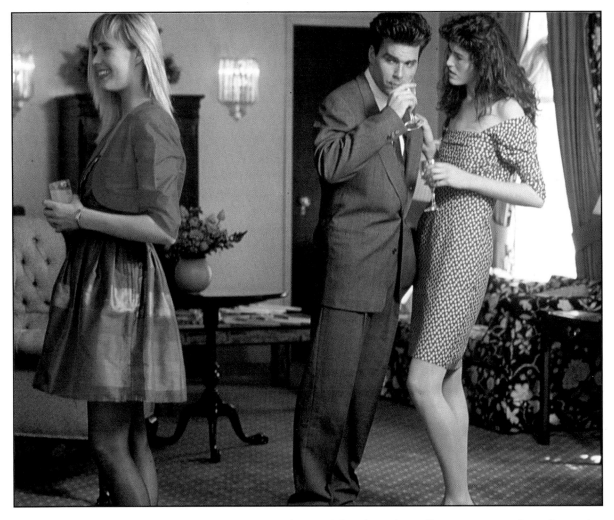

A lot of men like the idea of group sex—they fantasise about having two women make love to them.

nipples for a sexy tingling sensation that is immensely arousing. Plenty of women find orgasms easier to reach if a vibrator is used during lovemaking, either held by themselves, their partner or both.

Some men do feel threatened by them so any woman who likes to use a vibrator should try to be open rather than secretive about its use. Give it a name like Willie and treat it as a sexy weapon you share for extra bedroom fun.

GROUP SEX

Jenny was horrified when Alan suggested getting her friend Cindy to share a sex romp with them. "I once made the mistake of telling him she and I shared a bed when we were on holiday and ever since then it seems to have been on his mind. He said it would be fun for all of us as we're such close friends. I told him absolutely not but then he said how would I feel about doing it with a girl from his work who fancied him? I said no way as the idea turns me off completely. But he won't let it go and keeps trying to talk me into it. Now I'm wondering if I should just try it once to shut him up."

A lot of men like the idea of group sex—they fantasise about sharing their wife or girlfriend with another man or about having two women make love to them. Or about watching two women caress each other. They can be persuasive about this, so women often agree to threesomes against their better judgement.

Whatever the thrills, it is most likely to end in tears with jealousy, anger and guilt rearing their heads. A broken or damaged relationship is almost inevitable. This seems to be a sex game not worth playing, even if both partners are willing.

CROSS-DRESSING

Carol was gobsmacked, to put it mildly, when she found a pair of large-size black patent stilettoes at the back of husband Geoff's wardrobe. She guessed straight away that no woman had worn them: "They had to be his. I felt sick at the thought but I had to ask him about it. I found he'd been secretly wearing women's clothes for years. I couldn't believe it because he's such a masculine type, a big build and nothing feminine about him at all. Besides, our sex life was pretty good and he certainly showed no signs of being attracted to other men. I fell apart at the thought of him in a dress, I couldn't cope with it at all. He wanted to talk about it but I couldn't bear to hear, and I didn't want him to touch me. I felt our marriage was over because he'd been living such a lie."

But Geoff pleaded with Carol to stay with him if he sought help. They went to a marriage counsellor at first and then Geoff found out about an organisation that helped men deal with their need to dress as women.

Carol says: "I do understand now that Geoff's desire to dress up is not to do with

wanting to be a woman or with being gay. He says he feels better about it now that I know and am coming to terms with it. Now I've recovered from the shock of finding out, I realise that of course I do still love him and there's no way I'd let it affect our marriage. We've also met some other lovely couples in the same situation and it helps to know that there are so many other people out there doing the same thing. Now I even enjoy the fact that it clearly makes him so happy."

Plenty of women would run away from a cross-dressing husband because at first it may not seem an easy problem to understand or deal with. It is believed to be some men's answer to stress—they find that becoming a woman for a while relieves them of the pressures of their male roles. They can shrug off their responsibilities as providers, parents, bosses, leaders and let their soft side take over for a spell.

ANAL SEX

Mal had once had a girlfriend who enjoyed anal sex so he suggested it to his wife, Alex, as a way of adding spice to a night of passion. Alex got upset because she found the idea frightening and perverse.

"It's illegal, dirty and that's how people get AIDS. I felt sick at being expected to enjoy such a disgusting act," Alex said. "How Mal could imagine I would want to do it, I don't know. He said I was being ridiculous and that lots of people did it and I didn't know what I was missing."

Alex's alarm was understandable because anal sex, illegal in Britain though practised widely in other parts of the world, is still a taboo. Many heterosexual couples practise it with pleasure, though there is a health risk due to the large amount of bacteria in the anus and the danger of tearing the tight anal muscles. It can also be painful and many women find the idea degrading. Anal sex is not a cause of AIDS but it is the sex practice most likely to transmit the disease.

That's because AIDS is transmitted via the blood and blood is often present in anal intercourse due to tearing of fine tissues.

Having said that, if neither of you is HIV positive and you're in a long-term relationship, no straying on either side, you can practise anal sex without the risk of AIDS.

It is still wise to be ultra-careful about it, however.

Don't put anything—finger, penis, vibrator—in the vagina that has been in the anus without washing it thoroughly in between.

Use lots of lubrication like KY jelly.

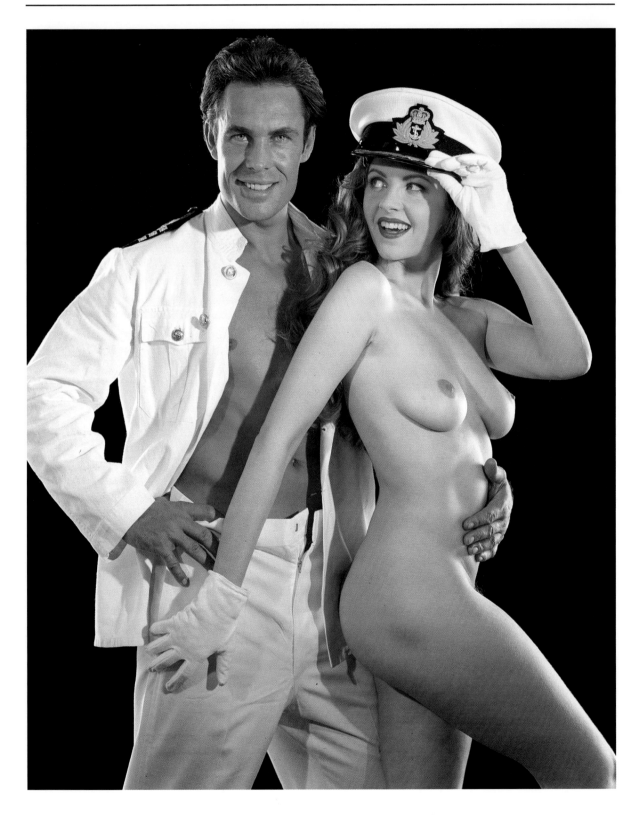

FANTASY SEX

How real can you get?

Like X-rated movies in which we are the major stars, our sexual fantasies flicker away in our heads giving us perfect love plots every time. No matter that we don't look like Kim Basinger, Julia Roberts, Mel Gibson or Tom Cruise, we can all dream, can't we? And when it comes to sex we let our minds run riot.

There isn't a red-blooded lover alive who hasn't experienced wildly uninhibited, daringly inventive, spine-tingling, perfect passion—all in the mind.

This is where we satisfy our secret desires, and fulfil the erotic longings we often don't dare mention. Here is where we become exotic love slaves, naughty nurses, swashbuckling squires and wickedly wanton French maids.

We also dream of being the object of Kim's, Julia's, Mel's or Tom's desire, having our wicked way with them, climaxing in an explosion of stars.

It's all very normal, say love experts, and does not mean that our sex lives are lacking. We don't necessarily want in real life the wild adventures we fantasise about—it's the thought that counts.

But acting out your fantasies with the one you love has become a highly-recommended way to spice up your sex life in an era when changing partners too often can endanger your health.

The hardest part is telling your mate that even though they're your Number One

lover, there is this other fantasy version you'd like to try out—if only they'd just slip into these thigh boots and leather gauntlets...

Your lover may, of course, be delighted at the chance to make your dreams come true. And they may have a few sizzling scenarios they'd like to try out on you, as well.

If that's so, feel free to indulge your fantasies till you run out of ideas. What you will find, almost certainly, is that the two of you will become even closer as you reveal your innermost sexy secrets to each other.

Even if you just titillate each other by talking through your fantasies—how you've always wanted to make love on the centre court at Wimbledon, how your mate has always longed to do it on a deserted beach at sundown—you'll enrich your love life with a new understanding of each other's needs.

Swapping sex fantasies can be a turn-on that hots up your performance even though you may never act out the love scenes of your dreams. Women, in particular, often find that filling their heads with torrid fantasies can help them to achieve sexual satisfaction.

Try not to be afraid of shocking your partner with your revelations of saucy daydreams—if they don't like the idea of one love game, describe another. Go through your fantasies together till you find one you share or feel willing to explore.

If you feel your lover is unhappy about

making your fantasy come true, don't push it. And if you are not 100 per cent happy to fulfil your mate's sexiest daydream, say so. Reluctantly carrying out sexy acts can only lead to unhappiness.

There are some very common fantasies indulged in by both men and women that are *not* meant to be realised. For instance, many women dream of being taken by force and many men dream of watching other men making love to their wife or girlfriend. But this does not mean the women would like to be raped or the men want to see others making love to their mate in real life.

These fantasies—and others about causing or suffering pain—are mostly in the guilty thrill category. They are a way of dealing with our secret, deepest fears by simply facing up to them in our minds.

These are the dark fantasies that few people want to reveal, even to their lovers, and are almost certainly best kept locked in your head. Be assured, you're not a sex monster just because you're turned on by shocking thoughts. It's only if you try to turn your dreams into unacceptable reality that you will be in trouble.

Many people have other fantasies they would like to put into practice: secret desires they would like their lover to satisfy, if only they could bring themselves to ask. Often these sex thrills we long for are the sort of things that others do regularly, like enjoying oral sex in a parked car (but please *not* on the hard shoulder of a motorway—it's illegal); having a quickie in a shop doorway or doing it while wearing rubber clothing.

But we are often shy about admitting our dirty thoughts. If you're a respectable mother of two, it might be hard to tell your children's father you fancy the *idea* of being a stripper at a stag night. If you're a macho truck driver, you may lack the nerve to tell your wife you spend a lot of randy moments imagining yourself as a schoolboy losing his virginity to his headmistress.

You have to decide which of your fantasies you can risk describing to your mate, which you should keep securely locked in your head and which you'd like to turn into reality.

Here are some DO'S and DON'TS to help make up your mind:

DON'T bother revealing your dream of being treated to oral sex if you've ever heard your mate say the thought of it makes them want to throw up.

DO mention you've always wondered what it feels like to be tied up during sex games if your mate keeps getting the video of *Basic Instinct* for your Saturday night entertainment.

DON'T ever be tempted to tell your loved one that you find it adds spice to your love life to imagine you are doing it with their best friend.

DO keep it to yourself if you dream of gay sex, even though the reality may not appeal to you at all. Your mate will only be upset, as there is no way they can fulfil your fantasy.

DON'T mention you get randy at the thought of sex from behind with a total stranger whose face you never see. Your partner may never let you near a crowded train again.

DO bring up the subject of your fantasies by discussing letters to agony columns or stories in sexy magazines. You don't have to admit your personal quirk—but watch your partner's reaction when it's mentioned. If their eyes brighten and they blush slightly, they like the idea.

And finally, *never* let your partner know if, at crucial moments of passion, you shut your eyes and think of one of your exes.

Fun fantasies appeal to most people's longing to play games with their mate, to pretend they are the heroes and heroines of their own dreams.

It's all good, harmless fun—even if there are no Oscars for your performance.

Many people find their fantasy life difficult to discuss with their partner. One way of communicating some people find helpful is known as bookmarking: you find an erotic scenario that appeals to you in a book or magazine and mark it by slipping a bookmark between the relevant pages. Leave it on your partner's pillow or bedside table, so they will know they are meant to read it.

You may find the following stories of how some couples turned their fantasies into full-blooded reality a source of inspiration—perhaps you might even fancy bookmarking one to get your lover's imagination racing in the right direction.

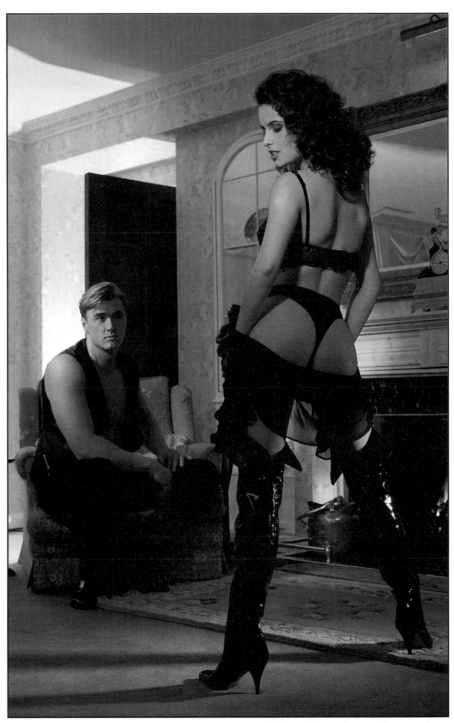

"One day I was having the usual thoughts about this girl on the train when I realised what I wanted more than anything was to see Sally doing a strip-tease, just for me."

Vince, a 28-year-old advertising salesman, always liked the idea of seeing girls take their clothes off, slowly, teasingly, like strippers.

"I'd see girls I liked the look of on the train to work and visualise them peeling off right there, dropping their skirts and stepping out of them in just their high heels, stockings and suspenders."

It was a scene he carried in his head, to cheer him up on the way to work. After he married Sally three years ago, Vince still kept enjoying his private strip-shows. Sally, a tights-and-bodystocking girl, is more inclined to strip off in seconds than stroll round flaunting her excellent body.

"One day I was having the usual thoughts about this girl on the train when I realised what I wanted more than anything was to see Sally doing a strip-tease, just for me."

Vince wondered how to ask his wife, since he strongly suspected she might laugh.

"I'd never told her about my fantasies—well, you wouldn't, would you? But one night I took the chance and told her about my favourite strip scene. She was very interested, to my surprise. She said, 'Would you like me to do that?'"

He admitted he would but she didn't say whether or not she was ready to make his day.

"I didn't think I'd mention it again. I didn't want to push her," he says.

He didn't have to. One night he came home to find Sally had set up a romantic dinner, his favourite steak in red wine, and was wearing something he'd never seen before, a slinky black suit with a long narrow jacket and a skirt that just seemed to wrap round her long, elegant legs. Unusually for her, she was wearing very high heels.

"Wow! what are we celebrating?" he exclaimed. She just smiled and said, "I thought you deserved a treat."

After dinner she led him into the living room where a fire was burning and she gave him coffee then went and sat in the big chair opposite him, carefully crossing her legs so her skirt parted, showing him a glimpse of stocking top.

"I thought I was dreaming," Vince remembers. "Then she said something about the fire being hot and started undoing her jacket. I noticed her boobs looked bigger and she had a cleavage I'd never seen before. She was wearing something black and lacy with thin red ribbons down the front of it."

As her jacket fell open, Sally lay back and raised one silky leg in front of her, admiring it as she let an immaculate black satin stiletto dangle from a toe. Then she ran a hand over one breast and trailed a finger down the dark hollow created by her uplifting bra.

"Like it?" she asked. Vince could hardly speak he liked it so much. He just nodded.

Sally stood up, walked over and put one foot on Vince's chair, slowly stroking the inside of her thigh. Then she turned and sauntered away, letting her jacket fall from her shoulders as she went. She tossed it across a chair and then started caressing her hips as she moved them slowly up and down. She unhooked her skirt and let it drop to the floor, standing there with her feet apart, wearing nothing but a curvy red and black basque, a satin G-string, stockings and suspenders.

"Want to see more?" she teased him, playing with the ribbons between her breasts, starting to undo the clips that would set her body free.

Vince stood up and walked slowly towards her. He wrapped himself round her and whispered, "Let's finish this in bed."

"It was fantastic," he says. "The best thing was, Sally loved it as much as me. We found we were both turned on by sexy underwear and the fun of stripping. It's not something to do every night but when we're in the mood, it's magic."

Shirt salesman Ronnie used to think the same saucy thought every time he saw his wife, Janice, scurrying round the house with the hoover or stretching up to dust the bookshelves.

"I used to try to think what she'd look like wearing nothing but a little frilly white apron and starched cap and black patent stilettoes.

"I fancied seeing her pert bottom in action as she flicked a feather duster about, like one of those maids in a French farce," says 44-year-old Ronnie.

He hadn't ever told Janice what was on his mind because he couldn't gauge her reaction.

"But one weekend our sons were going camping and she said, 'Let's do something we never get the chance of otherwise.'

"So I asked how she'd feel about being a French maid for the day—and she really got into the whole idea."

Ronnie could hardly believe his eyes on the Saturday when she brought him breakfast in bed.

"She had on a tight black basque, black fishnet tights and a white apron and her hair was pinned up with just a few curls hanging down from a little frilly cap. She looked gorgeous," he enthused.

"Shall I run a bath for *monsieur?*" she asked him sweetly as she teetered into their bathroom with a saucy wiggle.

Making sure he could see her from the bed, she bent over the bath to reach the taps, revealing that she wasn't wearing any knickers.

"She let me get settled in the bath then she came in and offered to scrub my back. She washed my hair then soaped me all over, leaning over so my face was pressed into her cleavage.

"I was tempted to let passion run away with me and pull her into the bath but I thought that would spoil the game."

At lunchtime, she set the table for one and told Ronnie: *"Bon appetit".*

"I pulled her onto my knee and told her to open her mouth while I popped a tit-bit in for her to taste. Then she did the same for me. We fed each other like this, finishing up with iced strawberries and frosted grapes which we washed down with champagne.

"I dropped my napkin under the table and asked her if she'd mind picking it up. She got down on hands and knees and started crawling under the long lace cloth, stopping so that all I could see was her gorgeous behind.

"I couldn't stop myself from touching her and next thing I knew she'd pulled me under the table and was tearing at my clothes."

Ronnie and Janice went to bed for the afternoon to recover. She put on the outfit again for dinner—and this time she ended up wearing it to bed where Ronnie made ecstatic love to her yet again.

"We both loved it," he says. "I'd never have believed Janice gave such an outstanding performance. She should have been an actress."

Every time Joanne walked through the park on a fresh sunny day her thoughts wandered in the same direction. How lovely it would be if Mitch was there, if we were that couple lying on the rug over by the big tree...

"I was always wheeling one of the children in a buggy and Mitch was at work on the other side of London so it always seemed an impossible dream," says 31-year-old Joanne. She would sometimes see couples locked together in the park and wonder if they were actually doing what she thought they were.

How could they? she'd ask herself—carefully looking away to they wouldn't catch her prying.

"Then I thought, hang on a minute, that's what most people do when they see couples who look like they're making love—

they look the other way. It's too embarrassing."

Mum-of-two Joanne then started wondering if she dared make her fantasy come true: "I thought about doing it in the garden but the neighbours would have a grandstand view. And it wouldn't have the same feeling of freedom, the same thrill of doing something outrageous right out there in the open."

She got her chance one weekend last summer when her parents took the children to the seaside.

"I didn't tell Mitch exactly what I had in mind because I didn't want it to feel too planned," she said. Her only preparation before heading for a nearby common was to wear a floaty skirt for extra modesty—and no knickers because it made her feel daring.

As they sipped chilled wine from paper cups she leaned over and kissed her husband and said, "Isn't this the best way to spend Sunday?"

"We could go home after lunch and make the most of having the house to ourselves," he said.

"Or we could just lie here and sunbathe a bit," she said, stretching out luxuriantly on the sweet-smelling grass.

Mitch rolled lazily towards her and started tracing the contours of her face with a long blade of grass. She undid one of his shirt buttons and started trailing a finger through his chest hair.

"There was no one in sight for miles so we just never thought about the risk. We just teased each other at first—he'd tweak my boob and I'd put my hand down his trousers, like kids behind the bike sheds. We were rolling round, laughing and playing, then suddenly he was on top of me and I could feel the urgency of his hand ripping his zip down."

This was the moment Joanne saw a family in the distance, moving towards them. "It was like all my fantasies, I couldn't stop what I was doing, Mitch couldn't see them so he wasn't bothered, he just kept on.

"So I just pressed myself to him as hard as I could and prayed they wouldn't come too close as my whole body went into wild spasms. Out of control. Out of this world...

"It was even more exciting than I'd imagined. I long to do it again as soon as summer comes."

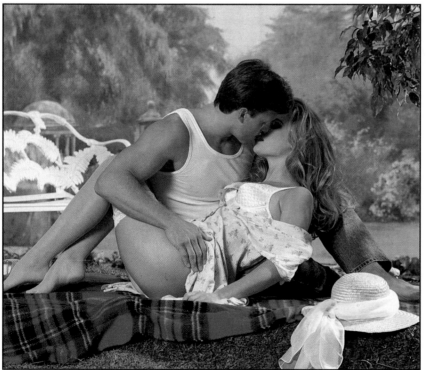

"It was even more exciting than I'd imagined. I long to do it again as soon as summer comes."

When she was a shy 17, Marea had been shocked when a man she'd just met on a blind date whispered in her ear: "I'd like to cover you in chocolate sauce and lick it all off."

"I thought it was the most disgusting thing I'd ever heard," says the 35-year-old hairdresser, married for 11 years to salesman Steve.

But she started thinking about the idea, what it would feel like, should the sauce be warm?

Marea began to have crazy flights of fantasy in which she featured as the Dish of the Day, being presented to a man seated on his own at a vast circular dining table being waited on by expressionless servants.

"They'd carry me in on a big silver dish and I'd be naked and sitting with my back arched, propped on my elbows with my head back.

"I'd have whipped cream spiralled over each boob, with a strawberry on top then there would be thin chocolate sauce in a lace pattern all over my torso and ruffles of cream circling the top of my thighs, like garters.

"Or I'd imagine I was covered in cucumber slices like a poached salmon, with lots of mayonnaise piped round my more interesting bits.

"The servants would all stand back and the man would tuck a big starched napkin at his neck and start to eat—without ever using his hands.

"He would do it very slowly, nibbling at the fruity garnishes and licking the cream and sauces very slowly and thoroughly so he got every bit. He searched every little crevice with his tongue.

"Then he'd put down his napkin and say to the servants, 'Thank you, you've excelled yourselves.'"

After Marea had been married about eight years, she got giggly over a few glasses of wine one night and confessed her fantasy to her husband.

"We had a good laugh and he said he could just see me as a game bird with the tail feathers sticking out of my bottom.

"But later in bed, he said he wouldn't mind trying the one with the whipped cream."

The next week they decided on a supper in bed, to be followed by Marea—as dessert.

"He loves trifle so I gave it to him a layer at a time—cake soaked in sherry arranged on my tummy, peach slices and strawberries tastefully arranged on gooey custard on my boobs, with cherries for nipples, and lots of whipped cream elsewhere.

"Of course I couldn't do it posed on a platter and Steve had to help with the serving, but it was brilliant.

"I kept thinking, if the neighbours peeked through the curtains now they'd think we were having some weird orgy," Marea says.

"I was being licked all over in the most delicious way and I could see Steve was enjoying himself hugely. He wasn't all dressed up with a napkin tucked in his chin, though. He was starkers, like me."

Since then, Steve and Marea have had a few similar bedroom feasts—some with her enjoying tasty morsels served off her husband's nude body.

"I used to think eating out was a major treat but now I know I can have a five-star feast at home with the kind of afters I used to daydream about, it's taken the edge off being taken out to dinner," she says.

"Now when I see amazing dishes in magazines or cookbooks I show them to Steve and ask, 'Could we do that one?'

"We have a great time imagining how we'd serve it up and who'd eat it off whom.

"It certainly beats sitting at the table with knives and forks."

Gary and Mandy always had a great relationship. After 15 years of marriage, the 41-year-old shop manager and his 37-year-old wife were the best of friends and their sex life was still energetic if not that varied.

"I suppose it was reaching the big four-O that did it but I began to feel the need for a bit more sexual excitement. I wanted to prove to myself that I was still attractive to women other than Mandy," Gary says.

But when he thought of actually doing something about it, he pulled back.

"I didn't want to hurt Mandy, I knew we had something far too precious between us to risk losing it," he says.

But he found he was looking at other women and thinking, "What if? Would she let me make love to her? Just once maybe? Would she tell?"

He worried that he might do something foolish. But then he got the idea of pretending to pick up a strange woman, who would in fact be Mandy.

"I read somewhere about a couple who pretended to be strangers meeting in a bar. I told Mandy about it, saying that I kept dreaming of making love to strange women. She was doubtful at first but then she went along with it."

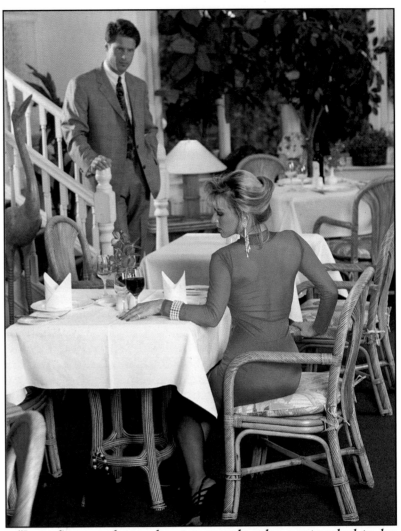

"I read somewhere about a couple who pretended to be strangers meeting in a bar. I told Mandy about it, saying that I kept dreaming of making love to strange women. She was doubtful at first but then she went along with it."

Mandy was perched on a stool with her back to him when Gary walked into the plush hotel bar. She wore a sexy red dress he'd never seen before, with a very low back.

"Are you waiting for someone or do you mind if I join you?" he asked politely as he stood beside her.

Mandy noticed immediately that Gary was wearing a new tie and smelled of an aftershave he hadn't used before.

"I'd like to buy you a drink," he said, looking admiringly at her new hairdo.

They sat, talking like strangers, flirting a little, over a couple of cocktails. Then Gary asked if she'd like dinner: "I know a little place not far away."

The restaurant was small and softly lit, with

pink tablecloths, fresh flowers, and a pianist tinkling in a corner. Mandy had never been there but the owner greeted Gary like an old customer.

Over dinner, Mandy noticed Gary seemed slightly nervous. He found her more animated than usual, she looked into his eyes more as she listened to him talk.

"It's been wonderful," he said as he helped her on with her coat. "How would you feel about a nightcap at my place?"

He walked her back to the hotel where they'd met and asked at reception for the key to his room, where chilled champagne was waiting in a bucket.

"Do you come here often?" she asked with a sly smile, letting her coat slide to the floor and kicking off her shoes.

He came over and ran a finger lightly down her naked spine. "I've been dying to do that all night," he said.

She shivered and he saw the hard outline of her nipples through the flimsy fabric of her dress. He pulled her to him to let her feel how much she had excited him.

"I'd like to undress you and carry you off to bed and have my wicked way with you immediately," he murmured.

"Please!" she protested. "We've only just met."

She pulled herself away, smoothing her dress. "Aren't you going to tell me your wife doesn't understand you?" she smiled. "By the way, how come they knew you so well at that restaurant?"

He grinned: "I asked specially that they greet me like that, to impress you."

"You think of everything," she smiled provocatively at him. "Let's go to bed and spend all night getting to know each other better."

Gary says: "That night proved to me that however well you think you know someone, they can always surprise you."

Wendy had once been in Palma, Majorca, when a naval ship was in port and she'd never forgotten how sexy the officers looked in their white uniforms, their gold braid and buttons glinting in the sunshine.

"There was something about they way they looked out from under their peaked caps that was both menacing and made me feel weak at the knees," she said. "I was only about 15 and they looked so powerful and in control. They looked the sort of men of the world who would sweep you off your feet and make you do whatever they wanted.

"I wanted to be crushed against one of those heroes' chests and have him tell me he'd look after me forever."

Wendy hoped for years that she might marry a ship's captain or an airline pilot. "I used to see films like *An Officer And A Gentleman* over and over, just drooling over Richard Gere. The thought of a hot-blooded male animal panting away under that perfect, starched white cloth literally drove me crazy."

Her husband, Roger, 35, is an assistant bank manager and the only uniform he's ever worn was at school. That was until they went to a friend's fancy dress party last year.

"I realised this was my chance to make love to a naval officer," says Wendy. "I told Roger I would organise the costumes and surprise him."

She hired a white naval uniform for her husband and, to keep it tropical, a Hawaiian grass skirt, bra top and flower garland for herself.

"Roger looked gorgeous. We'd just come back from a holiday and he was tanned and really looked the part. Women were coming up to him all night and telling him he looked fantastic. I got quite jealous because he was loving it," Wendy remembers.

When they were dancing, Wendy realised what it was about a man in uniform that made her feel so randy.

"I wasn't wearing much, so I could feel all the buttons and braid pushing against my bare flesh. It was making me shiver with excitement—I felt naked and vulnerable.

"What I most wanted was to get home and have him make love to me like one of those strong, silent heroes who won't take no for an answer."

On the way home she stroked the inside of his thigh as he drove and said to Roger, "I want you badly. I want to know how it feels to be ravished by an officer, not necessarily a gentleman."

He stretched out his hand and searched for the bare skin under the grass skirt. "I hope this doesn't get tangled in my buttons," he said.

Back home, he led her to the bedroom, shut and locked the door and ordered her to take off her scanty clothes.

She pretended to do it reluctantly, never taking her eyes off his face, looking slightly wary. He leaned against the door and

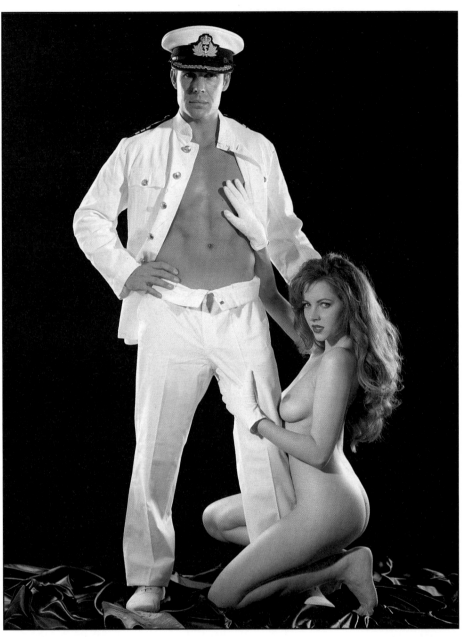

"I realised this was my chance to make love to a naval officer. I told Roger I would organise the costumes and surprise him."

watched her in silence, his hat low over his glittering eyes.

"I'd never seen him like that before. He was playing the part completely, loving every second. The moment I was naked he just walked towards me, took me by the shoulders and lay me down on the bed.

"Then he flung aside his hat, pulled off his shoes and fell on me, still fully clothed. We made love more frantically than we'd ever done before, as if he really had to say goodbye and go off and do his duty for Queen and country the next day."

Afterwards Wendy gently undressed her man and snuggled up in his arms to sleep.

"It was all I'd hoped for and more," she says. "I'm just waiting for the chance to do something like it again—Roger says he's ready to do it in uniform any time now he's seen what it did for me."

Whenever Gerry saw a sleek black limousine with tinted windows gliding through the West End of London he wondered what was going on in the back.

Obviously something that needed privacy.

"It's a turn on just thinking about it. Better than trying to do it in the back of a taxi with people going past in buses all looking down at you," he reckons.

Gerry, 34, a TV cameraman with a 30-year-old publicist girlfriend, Julie, liked to hope that one day he might be rich or famous enough to ride round in a chauffeur-driven limo in which he could enjoy daring amorous interludes.

Every so often they indulged in a spot of wild petting in the back of a black cab but they always agreed it wasn't the same.

Julie was used to hiring cars for superstar clients so she decided on a birthday surprise for Gerry. She'd turn up in a black-windowed Bentley to pick him up from work and they'd go home the long way.

"Don't drive to work today. I'll pick you up at seven," she told him on the morning.

When Gerry stepped out of the studio building on the dot, there was a uniformed driver by the door of a shiny black Bentley. He was astonished when the man said, "Your car, sir," but realised it was indeed

meant for him when the door opened and he saw Julie smiling in the back.

"She looked like a star. She was wearing a big fake leopard coat, huge dark glasses and her hair was cascading over her shoulders instead of tied back how she always wore it. I almost forgot to kiss her, I thought I must be hallucinating," says Gerry.

"A birthday drink, darling?" Julie offered, leaning forward and opening a gleaming walnut cabinet which turned out to be a fridge full of bottles. She swung open another door and reached for a pair of champagne flutes.

As they cruised along the bank of the Thames with the sun starting to set, they toasted each other and Julie said, "May all your fantasies come true tonight."

She was wearing a very short skirt which had ridden up as she slid back into the deep cushioned seat. Gerry noted her smooth brown thighs above black lace stocking tops. He let a straying finger stroke the inside of her thigh.

"Are we heading for Hyde Park Corner?" he whispered, leaning across to give her a lingering, champagne-flavoured kiss.

Behind the darkened windows they felt safe from prying eyes and even their driver was separated from them by a glass screen.

Gerry had his hands inside Julie's coat and was exploring every inch of her thinly-clad body. She didn't seem to be wearing anything besides a skimpy silk dress and the tiniest pair of lace bikini pants.

Together they slid down into the sensuously soft leather of the seat and while the peak hour traffic swirled by on either side their bodies melted together in blissful, uninhibited passion.

Gerry says: "There was something so erotic about being close to crowds in such an intimate situation. Now, whenever we feel like a real thrill, we order a car to take us across town and back."

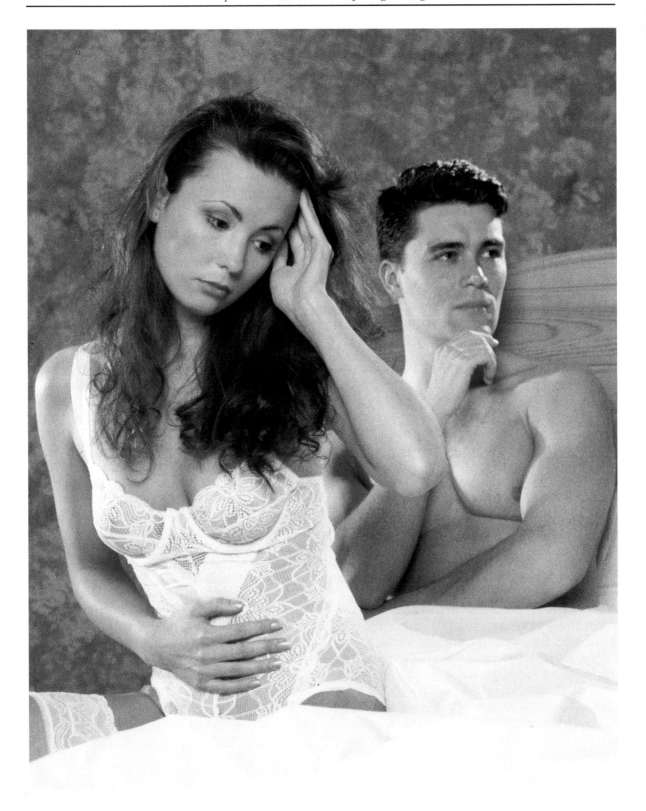

BEDTIME MANNERS

Animal passion is OK—but don't be a pig

Whether you're just on kissing terms or close enough to share your bed and body with someone else, you may be tempted to think that whatever you do will be acceptable to them.

That is, they won't mind if you pick your nose, scratch an itch or pass wind in their company. Take-me-as-I-am is your attitude and that's fair enough—as long as your lover isn't too sensitive.

But we all like to have our feelings considered, especially by the person we love most. And some of us can be touchy on the topics of sex, manners and personal habits. Even if you love someone to bits and you're sure there are no barriers between you, you still need to be aware of little things that might offend them—or turn into big problems if left unmentioned.

So here is the Supersex Guide to Sexual Etiquette which won't let you down when you're all steamed up.

It's so basic, it seems too obvious to mention *but* ... keeping your body clean, fresh and sweet-smelling will endear you not only to your mate but everyone else who is close to you. Not that you should drown yourself in perfume or after-shave, since the natural odours of men and women are more of a turn-on to the opposite sex. Just be aware that it's the natural odours

of *clean* men and women that bring out the beast in their lovers.

Since we're on personal hygiene, regularly cleaned and dentally checked teeth are a must if you want to stay kissable. No matter how gorgeous you look, a thick cloud of bad breath wafting from your mouth will send lovers reeling away from you.

Sex on a first date is up to you—thousands do it, though it's possible quite a few regret it when they sober up afterwards. Unless you're into living dangerously, it's madness to have sex with a stranger without using a condom. At worst they may be an HIV carrier and otherwise they may have a sexually transmitted disease like herpes—none of which will do wonders for your love life if you get infected.

Sex and drink are not brilliant bedmates if the drink is alcoholic and you have too much of it. It can certainly take the power out of a man's performance if the dreaded 'brewer's droop' stops him rising to the occasion. Women, without an erection to lose, lose their judgement instead and sleep with people they'd otherwise run a mile to avoid. You need to know how many glasses make you nicely uninhibited and how many make you legless—and stick to your limits.

Be nice to virgins, there aren't many of them about. If you are making love to someone who hasn't done it before, be gentle and try to make it a memorable start to their love life.

If you're about to lose your virginity, tell your partner it's your first time. Then they will know they have to lead the way.

Kissing is perhaps the most intimate pastime of all—prostitutes who will do anything else with a customer often refuse to kiss because it's something too personal to share with a stranger. So if you're just getting on kissing terms, don't start by thrusting your tongue down to your lover's tonsils. Try popping just the tip of your tongue into their mouth for starters, to test how they react.

Condoms can be a tricky negotiation. Don't wait till you're both panting with lust and tearing at each other's undies before you bring up the subject: establish that you'll use either a male or female condom—and that you've got one—as soon as it's clear you're going to bed together.

She will keep him in a state of excitement if she puts the condom on him when the moment arises. If she can do it with her mouth, it's even more tantalising. Practising this advanced skill with a cucumber is said to be helpful. (Or a courgette!)

Orgasms don't have to be simultaneous—though that's magic if you can get your timing right. But concentrating on your own as well as your lover's orgasm can be a bit like juggling oranges—one slip and your hands are everywhere, trying to make up for it. It's better to relax and not get frantic if you're hitting the peak of pleasure while your mate is still on the nursery slopes. Just be sure you stay awake long enough to ensure their satisfaction after you've had yours.

Your past is your business so keep it to yourself. Your lover may try to wheedle out of you whether they are the best bedtime fun you've ever had—but don't be lured into making comparisons. And don't give away the between-the-sheets secrets of any of your old flames. You wouldn't like them telling the world your sexy secrets, would you?

Flirting with others to tease your partner is okay if everyone knows it isn't serious. But it often turns out to be not such a brilliant scheme when everyone gets the wrong idea and someone ends up being hurt.

Putting your partner down in public is unkind and unwise if you want them to be loving and happy in private. On the other hand, making them feel good by praising them and telling others about their successes rather than their disasters will give you an ever-loving mate.

Say "I love you" to your partner at least once every day. It may seem corny and contrived but there's no one alive who doesn't thrill to those words. Only uttering them when you feel the urge to make love is *not* endearing—sounds more like persuasion than heartfelt emotion.

Kiss your loved one every time you come home and go out. Kiss good morning, goodnight and any time in between. Same goes for hugs and cuddles. Reserving your smooches and squeezes as preliminaries for wild passion is depriving your mate of affection. Both men and women need to feel loved without automatically being pounced upon.

A lot of men find it a job to know when their lover has reached the heights of ecstasy. If she hasn't screamed "Yes, yes, now, now, don't stop" or something similar and thrashed about a lot, they wonder whether they've done the right thing. But, please guys, don't ask, "Was that all right for you?" You might tempt her to tell you, "No, it was bloody terrible."

To help her man feel that he *is* Superlover, a woman can ease his worries by giving him a clue that it *is* all right for her. If she lets him know when she's about to reach orgasm, he knows he can go for it too. And "Mmmm, that was wonderful" is all she need whisper as she gets her breath back afterwards.

Telling your partner what you'd like him or her to do to please you in bed is the best of all ways of getting maximum pleasure. But do it nicely—don't say, "No, you fool, move it up not down," or "How many times do I have to tell you where my clitoris is?" Say, "Yes, darling, that's how I like it" or "Could you put your hand here for a bit?" A few contented sighs and moans helps things along, as well.

Ask what your mate would like you to do. Ask, "Is this nice?" or "Do you like it when I do that?" or "What could I do right now to make you really happy?"

Don't ever compare your mate's performance with an earlier lover. It's not a competitive sport and nobody wants to hear about their predecessor's ball skills or scoring tactics.

When you're in each other's arms and it's getting towards earth-moving time, don't shatter the moment by suddenly mentioning the leaking roof, the gas bill or what's going on in *Neighbours.* At least let your mate think you've got your mind on the job in hand

Talking about your partner's sexual prowess (or perhaps lack of it) to others is not doing anyone any favours. Your mate would never forgive you if they found out. Most people get embarrassed if told intimate secrets they know they shouldn't hear—so no

one on the receiving end would tell you so much as their star sign ever again. In short, anyone who dishes the dirt on a current lover Can't Be Trusted.

You might titillate your friends by telling them all the sordid little details of your sex fantasies. But don't let your lover down by revealing their fantasies to anyone, ever. Even after it's all over between you. Think how you'd feel if half the world knew what sort of thoughts turned *you* on in quiet moments.

It's a fact that men usually feel more zonked after sex than women do. *He* can happily roll off and be snoring with a smile on his face even before he's had time to say, "How was it for you?" *She* will feel quite glowing and exhilarated and want to be petted and snuggled for a few moments, to be reassured that she's really loved. So don't leave out the afterplay, guys. It only takes a minute.

Both men and women get headaches, bad moods, feelings of stress and depression, illness and other reasons why they might not be immediately ready for lovemaking when you offer it. So be prepared to take no for an answer if your mate occasionally tells you they'd prefer an aspirin to your advances.

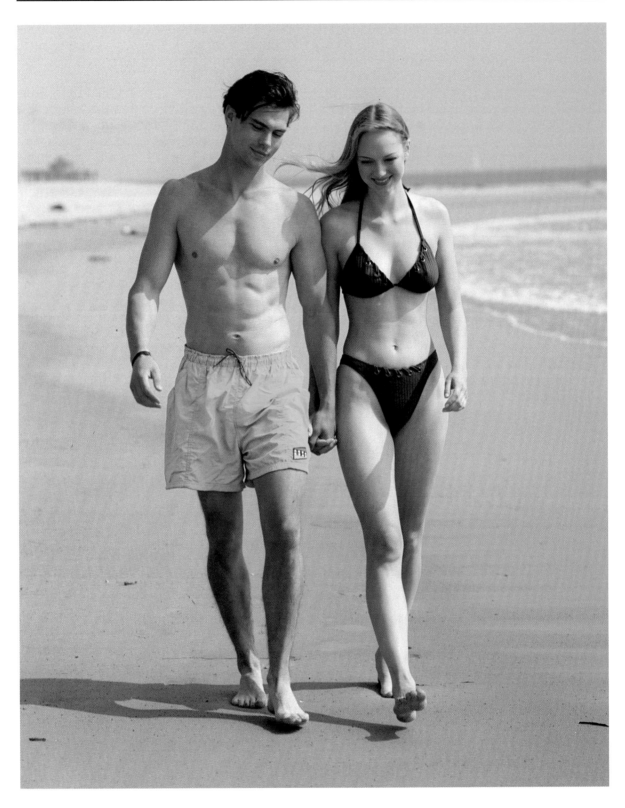

HOLIDAY SEX
When the lovin' is easy

You're far from home, the sun's shining and you're wearing little more than a smile. With your worries on hold for a week or two, no wonder you feel frisky.

Holidays can turn even the most cold-blooded of us into sex maniacs, whether it's our permanent partner in the hotel room with us—or a stranger sharing a short-term romance.

For wild, uninhibited sex, doing it in another country—or even another corner of Britain—is hard to beat. You're relaxed and ready for adventure, there are no nosey neighbours to spot what you're up to—and, if you've gone solo, you can love 'em and leave 'em at the end of the hols.

It's easy to try new strokes with new folks— or spice up your loving with your regular mate. For once, there's all the time in the world...

HOT HINTS

Stretched out on a sunbed with a drink and your long-term—or latest—lover, you'll feel randy stirrings rippling through your sun-kissed body.

If you're somewhere private, you can just roll over and satisfy your lust. But beware of sleeping off your sexhaustion where you lie—sunburn on your tenderest parts could ruin the rest of your holiday.

Rouse your mate to new heights of ecstasy with the way you apply their suntan oil. Linger over their most sensitive bits with loving fingers, then let them do the same for you.

You can do more with ice cubes than just cool your drinks. There's nothing more titillating than being stroked all over with an ice cube when you're feeling hot. Or being kissed by someone with a mouthful of ice.

Feed your lover ice cream from your breasts—or other interesting bits

Travel light, save washing and stay cool— by leaving your knickers at home. Specially if you're in a country where you have to keep your arms and legs covered in public.

Nude sunbathing on a secluded balcony or terrace can be a total turn on—and all bums look prettier when they're golden brown.

Lay off drinking exotic cocktails by the gallon if you want to enjoy a long night of love—the only thing less sexy than feeling sick is being sick.

When there's all day to make love, why not take all day? Hang out the Do Not Disturb sign and don't leave your room till dusk.

TRAVEL COMPANIONS

If you're not holidaying with your lover, who's your best travel mate?

If you go alone on a club or group holiday, you might have to share with a

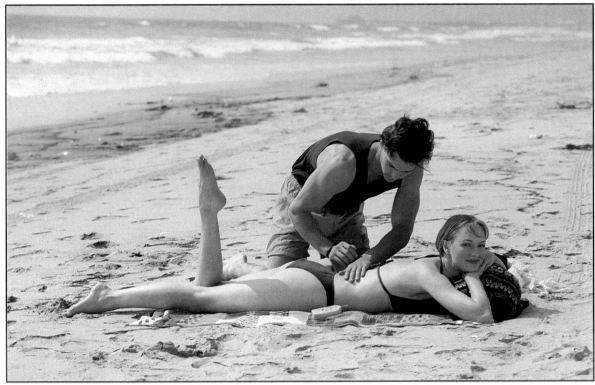

Rouse your mate to new heights of ecstasy when you apply their suntan oil. Linger over their most sensitive bits with loving fingers, then let them do the same for you.

stranger. So bringing someone back to your room could prove difficult—especially if your room-mate has the same idea.

If you go with a good friend, be sure you share similar views on holiday sex. If you're only interested in finding a lifetime partner and they fancy a daily fling with a different person, you may not be speaking by the end of two weeks.

Glenys, 35, twice-divorced, thinks a holiday without sex is like champagne without bubbles—flat and disappointing. She says: "Where's the fun? You only go away once a year, you've got to make the most of it. From the minute I'm on the plane I'm on the lookout.

"I've had a few drinks with a bloke on a flight and ended up in his room on the first night bonking my brains out. We've started on the bed, which was a single, ended up

on the floor and not even noticed till his mate tripped over us when he tried to get to his bed.

"It's all good fun, nothing serious. I've been around too long to hope I'll find the man of my dreams perched on a bar stool in Magaluf or Corfu. Better to treat them all like buses—if you miss one, there'll be another along in ten minutes.

"The worst holiday I had was with a girlfriend whose boyfriend had dropped her. She wasn't interested in having fun, all she wanted was to fall in love again. She thought I was disgusting for sleeping with people I knew I'd never see again.

"I told her, that's the point of holiday affairs—you don't particularly want to see them again.

"One chap did turn up once—and the magic had well and truly worn off. He was such a hunk in his swimming trunks larking about in Ibiza—but *so* boring in his grey work suit back in England. I'd rather not have seen that side of him."

WHAT TO PACK
• A phrase book with more useful lines than, "Where are the Roman ruins?"
Like: "You've got the cutest bottom on the beach"; "Tell me if you like what I'm doing"; "Stop—I can't bear it—you're hurting"; "OOoooh, do it again. Now. NOW."
• A rude book—to inspire steamier love-making.
• A torch—to light your way to the sand-dunes at night.
• A year's supply of condoms—in case the village shop runs out.
• A spare toothbrush—so you won't have to lend yours.

WHERE TO—AND WHERE NOT TO
Being away from home brings out the daring in all of us. Couples who've never ventured beyond the bedroom get the urge to make love on trains, boats, planes, beaches—and at famous tourist spots. And adventurous singles try to pull love-mates every chance they get.
Lovers reveal their top—and bottom—hotspots for holiday hanky-panky:
YES: Cross-Channel Ferry. John, 25: "My mates bet me I couldn't score before we hit France. Jane was with her sister who was seasick, so I gave her some travel pills and found her somewhere to lie down. From then, it was too easy. Me and Jane had a few bacardis then found ourselves a dark corner on the deck. It was cold so we were all cuddled up when I asked her if she fancied joining the Wave High Club. She thought it was a real laugh, doing it at sea. Being rocked by the waves is sexier than doing it in the air, I reckon."
NO: Where the tide may come in with a rush. Cheryl, 40: "We were in this tiny cove

at sunset, the most romantic setting. We were behind a rock making passionate love and didn't see the water till it swirled right up to us. We couldn't get back to the path and spent half the night shivering on a ledge."
OUCH: On the sand without a beachmat or towel under you. Sharon, 28: "We couldn't wait to get at each other. We'd had a few drinks so we went on the beach and got down to it. Talk about feeling the earth move—I could feel every little granule grinding into me as we rolled on the sand. It got in every little crevice. I had sand in my knickers for days."
OO-AH: In a public park or on a public beach in daylight. Ian, 31: "We thought there was no one round—or not near enough to notice. Next thing two police were stood over us shouting and there I was with my trousers round my ankles. Nothing you can say to that. We were lucky not to get arrested."
YES: In someone else's hotel room. Darren, 27: "We went to her room for siesta. It was cool and quiet and after we'd showered we smoothed after-sun lotion over each other and lay on the bed. It was hot as hell so we made love slowly, sipping icy water and drizzling it on each other's skin to stay cool. We made it last all afternoon."
YUK: In your holiday companion's bed. Mandy, 24: "I didn't mind that my friend brought this boy back to our room. I just went out. But when I got back I found they'd done it on MY bed. She said she was too pissed to notice. Well, thanks a lot, I think that's the pits."
YES: In a sleeping bag. Corrie, 29: "We met on the boat to the island. Neither of us could find a room that night so we went to the beach. He didn't have a sleeping bag and there was a cold wind so I took pity. We didn't do anything that night but by the next night I'd decided he was gorgeous. We undressed and slipped into the bag and

feeling the heat of his body against mine was all I needed. We made love and slept and did it again at dawn. Heaven."

YES: In your tent. Alan, 37: "There's nothing like it—you're private but you can hear all the sounds of the outdoors around you. It brings out the caveman in me—I like my women wild and earthy. My girlfriend does things to me in a tent she'd never do at home. She really lets loose."

MAYBE: Airport loos. Denny, 42: "I thought it was the last time I'd see her so I wanted to give her a proper goodbye. She smuggled me in to the Ladies and we did it in a loo while women came and went outside. It was definitely worth the discomfort."

OH NO: In a museum, palace or gallery. Eileen, 44: "We were going through this room with a four-poster hung with massive drapes and we both looked at each other and had the same wicked thought. We waited to hear no one was around then dived in behind the curtains. We were worried the bed would creak or even collapse so we did it rather gingerly, you might say. The hard bit was getting out afterwards. By that time we'd got the giggles and could hardly control ourselves—but we got away with it.

WHO WITH—AND WHO NOT

Holiday sex can be heaven or hell. Heaven when it's with someone you love on a balmy moonlit beach—and hell when it's a stranger in a foreign country who doesn't understand the word 'no' in any language. Rapes of British women holidaymakers in Greece should be a warning of the worst kind of nightmare—it isn't all like the plot of Shirley Valentine.

You need to be aware enough of local customs and culture to know, for instance, that a bra top and lycra mini may turn the locals into sex beasts if you wear it anywhere outside your hotel room.

You may be a nice girl who wants to go no further than sharing an ouzo and a peck on the cheek with the off-duty waiter—but your clothes will persuade him otherwise. Check local dress codes—and, for safety's sake, don't flaunt them.

Here's what other holidaymakers reckon about who to bed abroad:

BRITS IN SUMMER JOBS. Wendy, 26: "Kevin was a dream lover, so romantic. He seduced me on the deck of this yacht he was minding. It was just us on board and he took his time—easing me out of my bikini, kissing me all over, stroking and blowing gently on my wetted skin. It was heaven and it was like that every day till he put me on the plane home. I was warned he had a new girl every fortnight but you always think you're different. I thought this was true love. It was only later, when I didn't hear from him again, I knew I'd been used. I was just a brilliant perk of his job." *Rating: Fun! They can show you a good time—but don't expect it to last.*

FELLOW TOURISTS. Mark, 23: "I slept with a girl the first week in Majorca—I fancied her friend but one of my mates got off with her. My mate and the friend were together the rest of the time—and I got stuck with this girl who followed me everywhere like a sick dog. I couldn't get rid of her because we were in the same tour group." *Rating: Unadventurous—and they might follow you home.*

LOCALS MET ON THE BEACH. Annie, 19: "He drove me up into the hills and stopped the car, looking out to sea. Then he pounced. He was tearing at my top and climbing on top of me saying 'You want. You want.' I don't know how I fought him off and got out of the car. He just drove off and left me to walk back in the dark." *Rating: Everything your mum warned you about.*

HOLIDAY COURIER. Ben, 28: "She said she'd show me things most tourists never saw. We went to a deserted part of the island, a bay totally to ourselves. She said we didn't need bathers, so we stripped off

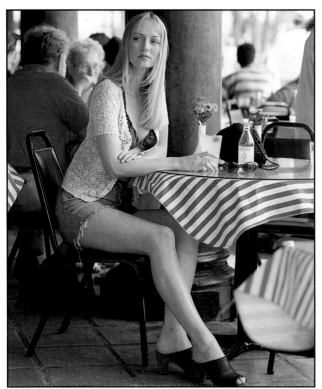

"He said he'd meet me the next night but he never showed."

and stretched out on the sand. Next thing, she was on top of me and her hands were everywhere. Then she started with her mouth and I thought I'd died and gone to heaven. We made love and swam and made love again—it was the best day ever. She had to work that night but she promised to see me again. I did see her, but only for a drink. She said she didn't have another free day till after I'd gone." *Rating: Nice one. No strings—but a great memory.*

LOCAL GIRLS WITH BIG BROTHERS. Don, 24: "She said no one was home during the day so she led me to her room and stripped down to just a gold chain and her big hoop earrings. She was like an animal, all over me, biting, scratching. We were just getting down to it when she froze and I saw her brother in the hall. She slammed the door and I legged it out the window. I was terrified her dad and brothers would come looking for me so I didn't leave the hotel for the rest of the stay." *Rating: Risky—unless you're with a lot of mates in the minding business.*

HOTEL MANAGER. Jenny, 38: "He was very smooth and he wouldn't take no for an answer. He knew I was on my own and he bombarded me with flowers, wine, chocolates. When he came to my door late one night asking to come in for a drink, I weakened. I thought in his job he wouldn't try anything. I was wrong. He wrestled me onto the bed and tried to make love. Eventually I talked him out of it and he left. I then spent the rest of my time avoiding him." *Rating: Thumbs down—he should be concentrating on his job.*

TEAM MEMBER. Rachel, 21: "He was there with his football team and we hit it off straight away. We spent the night on a sunbed down the beach and he said he never wanted it to end. He said he'd meet me the next night but he never showed. I saw some of his mates and asked if they knew where he was but they just looked embarrassed. I felt awful—as if they all knew and were nudging each other behind my back." *Rating: Iffy. Lads-together always put the team first.*

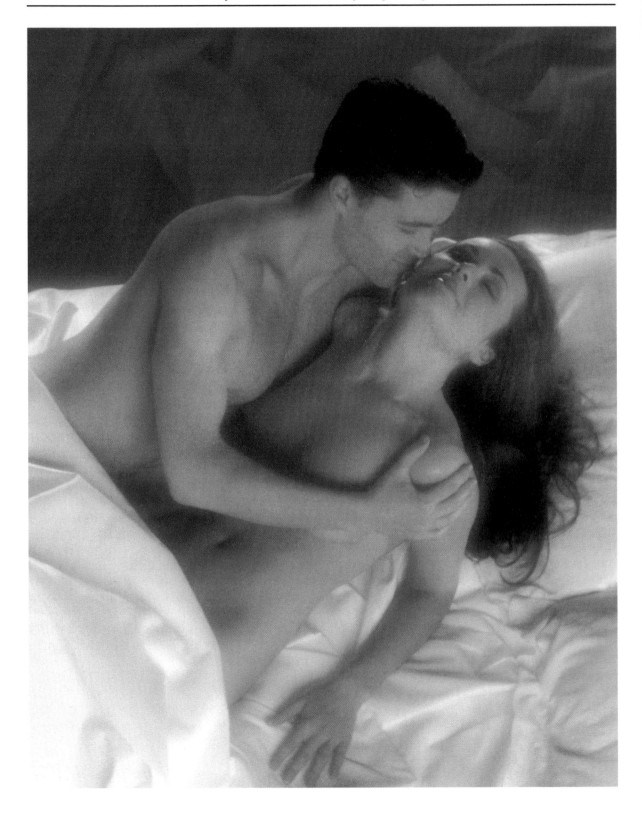

CONTRACEPTION
The pros and condoms

Now for the messy bit. If there's a downside of sex it's probably the worry of an untimely and unwanted pregnancy. Combine that with the fear of a fatal disease, i.e. AIDS, and you could sometimes wonder if it's all worth it: might celibacy be a hassle-free alternative? Or the DIY method (now we know it's normal, healthy fun and won't send you blind—see Chapter 1).

But then you think of the cuddles, the laughs, the all-night love-ins and there's nothing for it but to face up to the unavoidable necessities of contraception and, if you are not in a stable, exclusive relationship, safe sex.

As far as preventing the arrival of babies goes, there is a wide choice of methods, some far more reliable than others. If you're in a regular relationship the best way, by far, of sorting out the contraceptive problem is to talk it over together and decide what suits you both. Your health, religious beliefs, personality type—from fanatically cautious to incurably careless—all come into it. So do your priorities—if he refuses to wear a condom because it reduces his pleasure and she won't take the Pill because of possible side-effects, you'll have to come up with another idea from the methods available, which vary from the dodgy withdrawal method *(coitus interruptus,* you Latin scholars) to the mysterious inter-uterine-device (no one knows how it works).

It's a big decision, affecting the fun-level of your sex life, the happiness of your relationship and your future health and family situation.

If you're single and fancy free you have the added problem of safe sex to worry about. Is one night of passion worth risking your life for if you can't be bothered keeping condoms in your wallet or handbag?

To help you decide what to do to prevent pregnancy and stay healthy, here is the layperson's lowdown on the the pros and condoms of the methods available.

THE PILL
How: The combined pill, containing low doses of female hormones oestrogen and progestogen, stops eggs forming and moving to the uterus. So there are no eggs for sperm to fertilise. So you can't get pregnant. The progestogen-only, or mini pill, stops sperm entering the uterus, so it can't reach an egg, so you can't get pregnant.

What: The combined version is mostly taken one-a-day for 21 days, then you have a break of 7 days before the next 21-day stretch. The mini pill is taken daily and comes in packs of 28.

Pros: Nearly 100 per cent reliable—as long as a woman remembers to take them. The combined version keeps periods light and regular.

Cons: You need a prescription. The mini pill can cause erratic periods. Women who are overweight, smoke, are over 35 or have a family history of heart trouble or strokes would probably not be advised to take the Pill.

Who best for: Young, busy women in regular relationships who don't want to have to think about contraception every time they start to feel fruity. Also great for men!

Who worst for: Forgetful women.

THE COIL

How: The inter-uterine-device, or IUD, prevents eggs attaching themselves to womb lining but no one can explain why.

What: A tiny plastic object with copper wound round it. Has to be fitted and eventually removed by a doctor—but can last five years.

Pros: Reliable and if it suits you, worry free.

Cons: Messy, painful periods. Can lead to infertility as result of pelvic infection to which IUD users are often prone.

Who best for: Women who've had the number of children they set out to have but who don't want to be sterilised.

Who worst for: Childless women who hope to have babies in the future.

THE CAP

How: Seals off the cervix so sperm can't enter the womb.

What: A little rubber or plastic dome-shaped cap that fits over the neck of the womb. Has to be professionally fitted at first but can then be popped in and out when needed. Has to be kept clean and checked annually. Must be left in place for six hours after sex. Is much more effective if used with a spermicide which chemically sees off sperm in the vagina.

Pros: You don't have to keep buying them and there are no side-effects—unless users are allergic to rubber.

Cons: A bit unromantic and fiddly to have to decide in advance (a) whether sex is on the cards and (b) at what moment to reach for the cap.

Who best for: Women who don't have sex often and who fear side-effects from Pill-taking.

Who worst for: Women with false finger-nails which might get detached during insertion.

THE DIAPHRAGM

How: Seals off the vagina so sperm can't enter.

What: A rubber or plastic dome-shaped cap, larger than the cervical cap but basically the same. Its outer ring is outside the body, otherwise the technical details are the same as above.

Pros: Some women find the ring presses on their clitoris during sex and adds to the excitement.

Cons: A fiddle to fit and remember

Who best for: Gadget-minded women

Who worst for: Men who are impatient—or who can't hold fire

THE SPONGE

How: Makes it hard for sperm to survive the trip up the vagina to the uterus.

What: Circular sponge containing spermicide which is popped into the vagina before sex. Must be left in place for 24 hours afterwards.

Pros: Can be bought at any chemist. Some spermicides kill the HIV virus which causes AIDS.

Cons: Must be used together with another contraceptive like a condom, cap, diaphragm, otherwise there is a high risk of pregnancy.

Who best for: Women who are turned on by taking risks.

Who worst for: Couples with ten children and no spare bedroom

THE CONDOM

How: Prevents the man's semen making any contact with the woman's body.

What: A light-as-gossamer rubber sheath that encases the penis and catches the semen in a teat-like sac on the end.

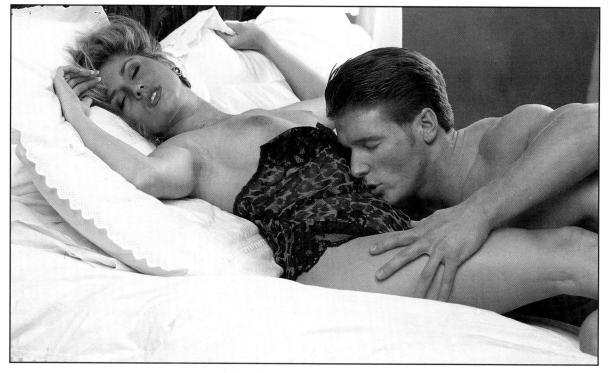

*The femidom can be inserted before the heat of passion
produces fumbles and carelessness.*

Pros: As long as they don't split during use, they are very reliable preventers of pregnancy and protectors against HIV infection. You can get them anywhere—often free, as when you get them from Family Planning clinics. They prevent discomforts like wet sheets and liquid running down women's legs.

Cons: They CAN leak if they're past their sell-by date, have been left in the sun or someone's teeth or nails jag them. They can also slide off when a man withdraws from a woman without holding onto the ring at the top. And lots of men say they spoil their fun when (a) they have to pause to put one on and (b) having their penis wrapped in rubber makes them less sensitive.

Who best for: Women who don't like a mess to clean up afterwards. Anyone worried about their partner's sexual antics in the past. Anyone who enjoys one-night stands.

Who worst for: Men with butterfingers and premature ejaculation problems.

THE FEMIDOM

How: Lines the vagina so that semen can't reach the uterus. Thrown away afterwards, containing ejaculatory fluid.

What: A fine polyurethane cylinder with a ring at either end. The end which goes at the top of the vagina is sealed. The open end is outside the body.

Pros: Like male condoms, they protect against HIV. Unlike the male version, which has to be put on the erect penis of its therefore excited owner, they can be inserted before the heat of passion produces fumbles and carelessness.

Cons: Inserting them can be a struggle and you have to beware of tearing them on rings and sharp fingernails. Worst of all, if the penis isn't carefully guided into a femidom it can miss and slide into the vagina outside it.

Who best for: Women who like to be responsible for their own protection against pregnancy and infection.

Who worst for: The sort of women who can't open milk cartons and who always open cereal packets where it says Open Other End.

THE JAB

How: The hormone progestogen prevents eggs being released from the ovary each month.

What: An injection in the backside either every eight weeks or every 12 weeks, depending on the formula.

Pros: You don't have to carry condoms or remember to take pills.

Cons: Can make you put on weight or bleed irregularly.

Who best for: Women likely to forget about taking precautions every time they have sex.

Who worst for: Women who can't stand the sight of needles.

THE IMPLANT

How: The hormone progestogen prevents eggs being released from the ovary each month.

What: Six thin plastic tubes are placed under the skin of the upper arm by a doctor. They contain progestogen which they release into the bloodstream for five years.

Pros: Worry-free contraception for five years.

Cons: A bit tricky to remove if you decide to try for a baby. Can cause erratic periods. No protection against HIV or other infections. Long-term side-effects unknown as it's such a new method.

Who best for: Women who go for hi-tech everything.

Who worst for: Women who worry about the side-effects of everything.

WITHDRAWAL

How: He pulls his penis out of her vagina just before he ejaculates.

What: Willpower and skilful timing are the only ingredients necessary.

Pros: No drugs, no appliances, it's free and you don't have to think about it beforehand.

Cons: Dead risky. Not all men know when to pull out and some just lose control. Even when he does withdraw in time, he may leak a few drops into the vagina. And a few drops can lead to pregnancy.

Who best for: Mad gamblers and couples who want large families.

Who worst for: Everyone left feeling unsatisfied and frustrated by the experience.

RHYTHM METHOD

How: By working out when she ovulates each month and refraining from sex on two days before and after that event.

What: Can be done by thermometer, since a woman's temperature dips then rises at the time of ovulation. Or can be calculated by counting the days between periods and trying to work out the half-way point i.e. roughly 14 days before the start of the next period, which is about when ovulation happens.

Pros: Approved by the Catholic Church. No drugs, no appliances.

Cons: Takes a lot of concentration, self-discipline and agonising.

Who best for: Very controlled couples.

Who worst for: Anyone hopeless with figures.

VASECTOMY

How: Sperm is prevented from reaching the penis so a man can only fire blanks—i.e. ejaculate semen without sperm.

What: The duct which carries sperm to the penis is snipped.

Pros: It's permanent.

Cons: Only recommended for over-30s who already have kids.

Who best for: Dads over 30.
Who worst for: Divorced dads who remarry and want to start another family.

FEMALE STERILISATION

How: Eggs are stopped reaching the uterus, so cannot be fertilised.
What: The Fallopian tubes which carry eggs to the uterus are snipped or sealed.
Pros: It's permanent.
Cons: Only recommended for over-30s who don't want more children.
Who best for: See above.
Who worst for: Women who change their minds about wanting more children.

MORNING-AFTER PILL

How: If taken within 72 hours of risky sex, prevents a fertilised egg from attaching itself to the womb lining.
What: Hormone pills, two taken within 72 hours, two taken 12 hours after that
Pros: Almost 100 per cent effective.
Cons: Strictly an emergency method.
Who best for: Anyone who suffers a burst condom
Who worst for: Anyone who can't get to a doctor in less than three days after risky sex.

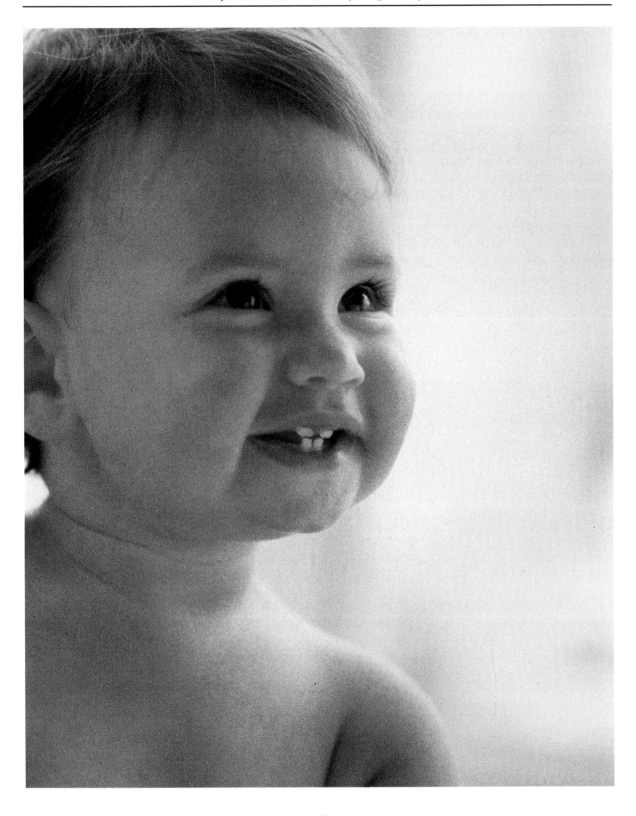

MAKING BABIES
How easy is it?

When you don't want to have babies, fertility is a curse to be fought off with contraceptives, self-control, celibacy even. But as soon as you decide you're ready for parenthood, it can still be a nightmare—if you happen to be among the fifteen per cent of couples who cannot conceive.

It's all a bit of a lottery. You do what you have to do to produce a pregnancy: that is, shoot several million sperm in the direction of the egg that one sperm alone has to fertilise. Then you hope for the best, in this case a missed period, to tell you a baby is probably on the way.

If you're a normal healthy couple who try baby-making two or three times a week, chances are you will succeed within a year. But if you try for a year without any luck, you'll then be off to your GP's surgery to try to find out why.

The first thing the doctor will check is that you're having sex in a way that makes babies possible—that his sperm is being deposited in her vagina and not in her navel, armpit or some other orifice. It's hard to believe, but in this day and age there are still couples who have not got the plot when it comes to sex. You who have read this book will know you are doing it properly, at least. What you may not know is exactly how chancy the whole business of babymaking is. You MAY hit the jackpot and produce a pregnancy in the first month of trying—there's a one in three chance of this among couples whose fertility is proven. But after that, your chance of conceiving each month drops to an average one-in-four to one-in-five. One in ten fertile couples takes more than a year to succeed and one in twenty takes more than two years.

You may then wonder how it's possible for the world to be so over-populated. That's because we are living longer and stronger, and has nothing to do with our reproduction rate which, compared with other animals, is fairly pathetic.

BABY BASICS

Here is what happens, from bonk to baby, if it goes like clockwork all the way:

An egg starts travelling from her ovary towards her uterus and is ready for fertilisation. This happens once a month, between periods.

You time it right and make love at a moment when the egg is on its journey.

His semen, containing literally millions of sperm, spurts into her vagina and the sperm start swimming like fury to get through the cervix into the uterus and towards the egg.

The sperm that make it cluster round the egg and one manages to fertilise it. The rest then die. Thirty-six hours later, the egg splits into two cells which then keep dividing till a ball of cells reaches the wall of the uterus and attaches itself there. This takes about four days from fertilisation.

About eight weeks from fertilisation, the embryo attached to the uterus wall has a sac of fluid surrounding it and has turned into a foetus with a head, arms, legs and recognisably human form.

Forty weeks from the first day of the woman's last period the baby is born.

RAISE THE ODDS

Some couples have more chance of becoming parents than others: the randier the couple, the more often they have sex, the more likely they are to start the baby process. You don't have to be a genius to work that out. But that is presuming he has a normal sperm count and she ovulates regularly.

A Norwegian survey of 252 men revealed that a man's sperm quality rose along with the number of times he ejaculated it. So men with a low sperm count who are often advised to refrain from sex to let their sperm count build, may be achieving the opposite result from the hoped-for one. The same survey found that, contrary to medical belief, sperm quality did not deteriorate if a man wore tight underpants, smoked, drank or sat soaking in hot baths.

But apart from trying more often, there are other ways said to improve your chances of babymaking. For instance:

Bring science into it. If she takes her temperature first thing every day and makes a note of it in her diary, she will notice that about midway between her periods the temperature will drop slightly, then rise slightly. This is the sign that ovulation has taken place—you then have between 12 and 24 hours of prime time to fertilise that egg.

Stop worrying and learn to relax. Women overcome with anxiety about motherhood and feeling pressured to reproduce often seem to have difficulty getting pregnant even when there is no physical reason to prevent it. It is believed that stress affects

the hormones which in turn interfere with the timing of ovulation. Men under stress may also be less likely to conceive.

So, if a relaxed and happy couple has a better chance of making babies, can you learn to stop worrying and start producing? You can try. Yoga, meditation, massage and other relaxation techniques can be calming for the mind and soothing for the body.

Don't go on a crash diet. Any woman who has lost a lot of weight in a hurry will tell you that it can cause chaos with the monthly cycle. Missed periods, stopped periods, totally erratic periods are frequently a side-effect of heavy-duty dieting. Putting on a load of weight won't do wonders for a would-be mum or potential dad, either, since that also throws out the hormone balance, making for sluggish loving and a drop-off of desire.

Don't take up strenuous exercise if you've always been a slob. While peak sports performers tend to be virile lovers, it's unwise to throw yourself suddenly into an unaccustomed fitness programme if you're trying to have a baby. Women who start running or working out, when the most exercise they've done since school is remote-control the telly, may find the shock of exercise plays havoc with their periods. That is, ovulation becomes unpredictable, diminishing chances of conception.

Stay cool. Sperm hate heat, scientists say. The temperature in which they survive best is two degrees cooler than the rest of the body which is why nature designed the testicles containing the sperm to hang in a sac *outside* a man's body. But tight jeans and snug underpants tend to hold the testicles against the body, raising their temperature—which tests have shown can reduce the sperm count. Loose trousers and boxer shorts are said to be best for male fertility.

Stay in bed after love. Once a man has done his bit and left his sperm to battle their way through a woman's cervix and on to find an egg in a fallopian tube, she can help the process by lying back with a pillow tucked under her bottom and knees up to her chest. This tilts her pelvis upwards, the theory being that it gives the sperm a better chance of making it through the cervix, helped by gravity. Anyway, it's quite a comfortable way to lie for half an hour or so.

Eat organic veg. Men who eat food which is free of pesticides have double the sperm count of those who don't—this was the finding of tests carried out in Denmark at a convention of the Danish National Organic Farmers' Board. So far, scientists are sceptical of these findings but there is increasing belief that pesticides, detergents and food additives may be responsible for the alarming fact that men are only half as fertile as they were 50 years ago. Research in 20 countries has confirmed this piece of bad news.

WHEN BABIES DON'T HAPPEN

We all presume we will be able to produce children when we want them, if not also when we're not actually planning to increase our families. So once we have thrown away the condoms, stopped taking the Pill and doing whatever else we did to prevent unwanted pregnancies, we expect to become mums and dads almost immediately.

If the months go by without success, we start to worry. Everyone else seems to have babies as easily as picking one off a supermarket shelf, so why not us?

If you're worried about your lack of reproductive success you will almost certainly consult your GP. He or she will probably tell you not to be impatient, it can take longer than you think. Surprisingly, it's quite normal for a couple to take three years to conceive—through simple bad luck rather than any problem at all.

If you're under 30, it probably won't be thought necessary to send you for fertility tests till you have spent three years failing to produce. But it's highly likely that, once

having talked your worries over with your doctor and gone away encouraged by the reassurance that It Can Take Longer Than You Think, you will find yourselves miraculously parents-in-waiting at last.

The famous American sexperts, Masters and Johnson, found that one out of eight couples who attended their infertility clinic over a 25-year period conceived within three months. And that was just as a result of being given the basic facts about chances of pregnancy and how to increase them.

If a woman is over 35, however, most doctors won't delay to see if nature can do the right thing. Her fertile time is running out so they may just get on with trying other possibilities such as Donor Insemination (DI) or In Vitro Fertilisation (IVF) which means fertilising the egg in a test tube before implanting it in her uterus.

Contrary to an old-fashioned belief that failure to conceive was usually the woman's fault, it is now established that it is equally likely to be the man's. And in nearly one-third of cases, it's a problem shared by both. So it is important always that both partners' fertility is put to the test, if it comes to that.

Lucy, now a 31-year-old mother of two, was convinced, when she started trying to get pregnant five years ago, that she would have her babies almost to order.

"All my friends were popping out babies as easily as rabbits and I just thought when I was 26 that it was a good age to start a family. I thought I'd have one by the time I was 27 and another before I was 30 and that would be it. Family complete.

"I planned to stop work at 7 months to get ready for the birth and perhaps, if we could afford it, to go back after our second was born. But it didn't turn out like that at all."

She and husband Tony grew gradually more glum as the months passed and no baby was on the way. "After 15 months it was getting me down. Every month I would pray I could chuck away my tampons, every day I calculated my period was late I would hope beyond hope. I got so miserable it was making Tony depressed as well—we couldn't think of anything else. At first we'd been bonking away cheerfully with the happy thought of the beautiful babies we'd be making. Then after a bit it started to feel like a waste of time. I think we were each secretly blaming ourselves and we got to the stage we could hardly talk about it, we were so screwed up."

That was when Lucy went to her GP and asked, "What's wrong with me?" She was cheered up to hear her problem was almost certainly no more than a spell of bad luck. "That and bad timing," she says. "I'd always thought that if you bonked regularly, you could scarcely fail to hit the jackpot. I wouldn't have dreamed of counting days and trying to pinpoint ovulation exactly. That sort of thing seems so calculating.

"What I never realised was that it can take more than two years to get pregnant—not surprising when you consider the very few hours in each month when it's possible.

"The trouble is, we all grow up being told you can get pregnant at any time of the month and without even bonking—all the scare stories to make you careful—so you think it'll happen in seconds as soon as you stop taking precautions.

"I went home and told Tony we were being crazy to worry so much. It seems ridiculous but I felt so much better after just talking to my doctor and getting the facts straight. She also gave me a load of advice on improving our chances which all seemed pretty sensible. Somehow it lifted the pressure we'd both been feeling.

"We celebrated our relief with a couple of glasses of wine, went to bed and, I know it seems incredible, I discovered I was pregnant about six weeks later."

Other couples are not always so lucky. It is estimated that 10 to 15 per cent of cou-

ples are infertile—though that includes the significant number who find they cannot conceive a second child.

The main causes of infertility are. . .

Ovulation failure: A sign of this is a woman's lack of monthly periods which may instead occur rarely or not at all. There are various causes and nearly all can be successfully treated—except for early menopause.

Tube blockages: Damage from a number of causes such as stomach surgery, appendicitis, miscarriage, childbirth or sexually transmitted infection can affect the tubes so they do not work normally. Surgery can remove blockages but chances of pregnancy afterwards are not very good. The test tube method of reproduction is said to be a better bet.

Sperm problems: Even men with a normal sperm count can have severe problems trying to father children if their sperm doesn't perform as it should. It's not the sperm count that matters, it's their performance. A man with a low sperm count can be fertile while a man with a normal count can be infertile, if his sperm is unable to survive making its way to the waiting egg. A test about 12 hours after intercourse can check on the progress of swimming sperm. If there is a sperm disorder, a couple's best chance of conception is said to be by donor insemination. Otherwise, they may prefer adoption.

Mark and Louise married when both were 35, after a first pregnancy which ended in miscarriage at seven weeks. They tried to conceive for about a year before seeking help.

"I had to go privately because the NHS waiting list was two years and I was already 38. That seemed to make little difference except that you paid much more. You were always kept waiting a minimum of two hours, saw the consultant for five minutes and he'd say come back in three months. This kept happening—I was having various tests which showed no problems, but nothing was being done."

Louise found herself attending a string of private fertility clinics. "Your morale goes up and down like a yo-yo. You keep trying then you give up for a while. Then someone says they know another doctor..

She went to one for donor insemination: "Just as I was rushing up the steps, this guy came shambling out and he had long greasy hair and was dirty and I thought, oh my god, is that my sperm donor?"

She was made ready by a nurse to receive the sperm. "The doctor was supposed to have specific details of Mark—height, colouring etc—but this nurse sat there, with the sperm, asking, 'Now—what does your husband look like?' She didn't know whether he was dark, fair, short, tall. All she could say was, 'I can't read the doctor's handwriting. But never mind.' And she closed the file and gave me the sperm. And you take it because you're desperate. But your imagination goes berserk."

She was then recommended to another:. "I went to this woman in Harley Street who was into douching with bi-carb soda. You have this bag you have to hang on the shower above you in which is a mixture of bi-carb and then at the right moment you have to douche—not more than ten minutes before the sperm is going to come inside you. Can you imagine? The only thing that kept us sane was Mark's sense of humour. I know so many men who would refuse to go through with it but Mark was absolutely wonderful. He always made a joke and got on with it.

"One morning he was ready for work and I took my temperature and there it was, the moment for action. So he took off the bottom half of his clothing, leaving his shirt and waistcoat on and we did it—and I got pregnant again." But for a second time she miscarried.

"Mark was inefficiently tested in the beginning and all the way along the assumption was that the fault was with me. It took a long time to discover that 50 per cent of his sperm were unhealthy and it's possible I miscarried because the egg was fertilised by unhealthy sperm. It took three years before we got an adequate analysis of Mark's sperm: a sperm count, a motility count (to check the sperm's movement) and one to check whether it's deformed or not. "They then put Mark's sperm in a spinner and only the good ones came out, the bad ones were left behind. Then they mixed the good ones with other donors' sperm.

"We had about six attempts at insemination with mixed donor sperm by which time I was 40 and my chances were getting slimmer. We started investigating IVF but the hospital said at my age it was only worth trying three times because of the cost and the low chance of success.

"But before we got to having the IVF treatment, we decided to adopt instead—something we had also been investigating all along."

They now have a five-year-old daughter, adopted in America.

"We both gave up on our bodies in the end. You keep trying while there is hope but in the end you can't keep going. It was a great relief when we stopped."

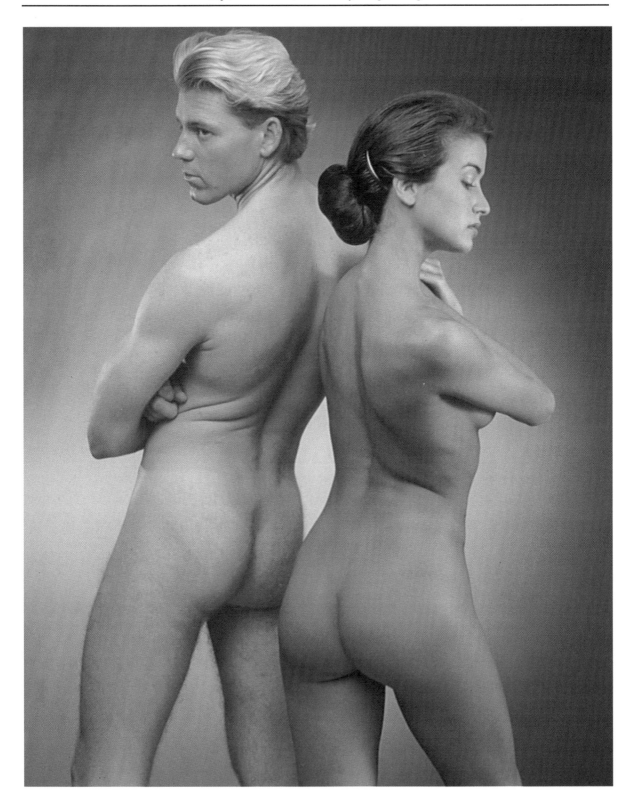

PROBLEMS
Too tired? Too busy? Too nervous?

Only in romantic novels do lovers fall into each other's arms and beds, in perfect sexual harmony from the first fizzing kiss right through to the first tumble onto the mattress—and, we're led to believe, for more-or-less-ever after. The heroines never have headaches and the heroes always hold fire till their partners are thrashing about in a wanton frenzy of readiness.

That is the ideal some of us think we'll achieve, given the right mate: a rosy-glowing sex life with never a hitch, never a night off.

The other common expectation is quite the opposite: bedtime will be a thrill-a-minute for about the first two years—then it will go downhill forever more as both of you turn off desire and switch on to other interests. Could train-spotting or ferret-fancying be better than sex, you may wonder?

Everyone expects something different from sex, according to what they know of it from their parents and families, from what they've read, seen and heard. So any pair of lovers may find, after a while, that each has a different idea of what makes a deeply satisfying sex life. *He* may think it is being able to have sex whenever he feels like it and *she* may think it is being wooed with wine and roses every single time. So when events don't match up to the ideal and either or both partners are not getting

what they want, the barriers go up at bedtime.

It is not always a sex problem that leads to frustration between the sheets. Whatever the aggro between a couple, from disagreeing over the household chores to differing over each other's friends, sex always seems to suffer. Someone withholds it, someone never feels like it, someone can't do it any more. And if a couple can't talk to each other about what's gone wrong, it will go from bad to disastrous.

Sexual distress is difficult to talk about—so problems often fester because no one knows how to mention them, let alone deal with them. One partner may think that, because they don't get stirrings of lust any more, the laws of nature have decreed the relationship over. Another may blame their mate for the dwindling of passion between them—while some downcast lovers will always blame themselves for a partner's lack-lustre performance. So defeat, anger, guilt, despair can all build up to grief and shattered relationships.

It need not be like that. Facing up to a problem when it's just a niggle rather than waiting for it to reach epic proportions is the key to keeping your sex life alive and well.

But how do you spot the problem? If your partner suddenly seems to have lost their enthusiasm, how do you know if it's because they've fallen for someone else, they're depressed about work prospects or they hate the fact they've put on weight? And how do you ask them, for goodness sake? "Have you stopped feeling fruity now you're fat?" If you want to kill off the relationship, attacking your mate for a problem *that you share* is a fast way of going about it. It should always be remembered that any problem between two people is a problem for both of you. If one of you wants to blame the other entirely, it will be almost impossible to solve. And if you choose to suffer in silence because you fear hurting your partner's feelings or making them angry you are committing yourself to a lifetime (or as long as you can stand) of resentment. Is that fair to someone you think you love, let alone to yourself?

Sex problems make us feel ashamed because most of us presume that everyone else is merrily bashing the bedsprings in everlasting bliss. We don't want others to know that our last three bonks were no-score fiascos or that we'd rather go to bed with a steaming cup of tea than a red hot lover.

The first thing to realise is that what other couples do is irrelevant to us. They will have their own problems from time to time which may or may not be similar to our own. Using what others do—or what we *think* others do—as a yardstick or trying to fit in with some imagined norm has only one likely outcome: problems. If you are happy making love once a week then learn that twice a week is the national average, worrying that you are less lusty than lots of other couples may start to spoil the sexual pleasure you have always enjoyed. The problem that starts in your head will end up in your bed.

Men who worry about the size of their sexual equipment, women who expect their men to 'give' them orgasms rather like handing them a piece of cake, couples with very different libido levels, can all agonise

their way to tears at bedtime.

But problems can be solved if you face up to them like the following couples did.

PROBLEM: Roger and Carol had a shaky start to their relationship in that he was recovering from the pain of a divorce, his ego damaged from being dumped by his ex-wife. Carol, 24, was anxious to reassure him and also to prove herself an exciting lover. "I suppose I was competing with the memory of his wife, trying to be better than her. And because he's eight years older than me and had had loads of affairs, I felt I might seem inexperienced and boring in bed.

"I did everything I could to turn him on and make him happy and didn't really think about me. His pleasure was all that mattered at first. He kept telling me I was fantastic in bed and that was all I wanted to hear."

But after a few months she started to realise that their lovemaking was leaving her with an empty feeling. Roger was a caring lover but somehow he'd always leave her high and dry, desperately unsatisfied.

"I didn't know how to tell him he wasn't giving me orgasms. I just got angry inside about it. Even when he'd ask me about what I liked him to do, I felt angry—I thought he should know without having to ask. Specially with his experience."

Roger sensed her dissatisfaction but couldn't get Carol to talk. She did, however, pour out her frustration to her best friend, an older woman. "She said I would never have an orgasm if I thought of it as entirely Roger's responsibility, something he could give me like a present. I had to find out exactly what excited me—maybe by trying out pleasuring touches on myself—and let Roger know what I liked and when to keep going with something and when to stop.

"She said I should tell him gently, as we made love, what I was enjoying and what I wasn't—but not like a criticism or a running commentary. More of 'Mmm, you can do that all night if you like' and 'Please darling, more of that'.

"She also said I had to be more selfish and learn how to concentrate on my own pleasure, lie back and let Roger take control for a change.

"What she said made me think differently about what was happening between Roger and me. I realised I was being unreasonable, expecting him to mind-read what I wanted him to do.

"It was quite hard, changing the way I'd thought about sex and trying to make things better for myself. But Roger seemed to understand and appreciate that I was trying. When he asked me what I wanted, I started being able to tell him instead of turning away in silence. Gradually, we worked things out between us and now I seem to have orgasms as often as I want."

PROBLEM: Tiredness and overwork were the problems that caused engineer Ted's sex drive to flag so badly his wife, Trish, was convinced he was being unfaithful.

"He was always late home from work, which I found irritating but I knew couldn't be helped. His job was demanding and the trip home took an hour.

"He'd have a quick drink and sit down to dinner, often hardly speaking because he was so knackered. Afterwards he might watch a bit of telly or read but it wouldn't be long before he was starting to nod off.

"Occasionally I'd try to stir him to action by climbing into his lap, feeling my way into his trousers and giving him the kind of treat that used to have him ecstatic in minutes.

"It would seem to rouse him momentarily but then he'd brush me away. He'd say, 'Please, there's no way, give us a break.' Sometimes he would really try, once we got to bed. But either he would pump away for ages till we were both exhausted and no one was having any real fun, then we'd have to give up.

"Or his erection would start to go limp before we'd got to the penetration stage and he'd mumble he was sorry, he wasn't in the mood.

"I was getting frustrated as hell but he didn't seem to think there was a problem. If I tried to talk about it, he'd sweep it aside."

When Ted started having the odd meeting at weekends, Trish decided he must be having an affair. She was hardly seeing him, when she did it

"I realised I was being unreasonable, expecting him to mind-read what I wanted him to do."

was fraught and she'd begun to have ideas of ending the marriage.

She confronted Ted with her fears and accusations and he broke down, shattered.

"His company was going through upheavals, he was fighting to keep things afloat and keep men in work and he just had no time for anything, let alone another woman. He was appalled that I'd thought it. It all came tumbling out then, including his de-

pression over his sexual failure and the fact he'd lost the urge.

"If only we'd managed to talk about it earlier. I felt desperately sorry for him, all my anger just melted away."

They decided Ted should see their GP for a thorough health check. Then he should take his first proper holiday in two years.

"We went to a remote hotel in the Lake District and just vegged out. Sometimes we'd stay in bed till lunchtime, then we'd walk or lie in the sun, nothing demanding. We enjoyed each other's company, had time to talk and cuddle and make love when we felt like it.

"We took things slowly at first—I realised that part of Ted's problems must have been from me grabbing at him and trying to get some action out of him before he fell asleep. Poor guy. But once we were away, with time to ourselves, the problems vanished.

"He was a new, lusty man in just a few days. I think it was also due to his decision to start planning ahead to leave his job and work for himself as soon as he could.

"He realised he was wrecking his life and probably his health by the way he'd been working. He decided that, for him, it wasn't worth it. I don't think he'd ever questioned what he was doing before. He thought there was no other option.

"One of our main problems was we'd stopped talking to each other but now that's all changed. We never stop. Ted also now makes sure he's

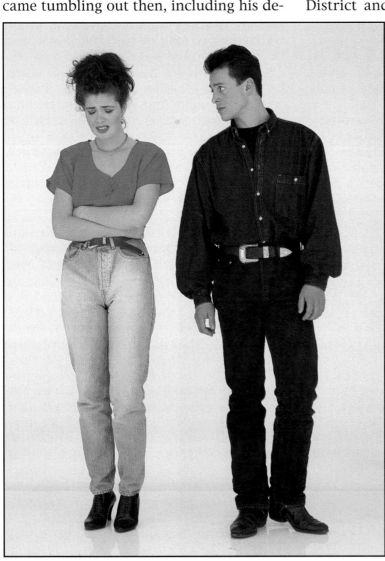

"When I asked him about the porno videos he got a bit shifty and said they were his mate's."

home early two nights a week—and he's taken up fishing at weekends."

PROBLEM: Fear and ignorance nearly destroyed Mick and Libby's two-year marriage after she found a box of porn videos in the boot of his car.

"When I asked him about them he got a bit shifty and said they were his mate's. I suggested we watch one and he didn't seem that keen, he said I might not like it," said Libby, 26.

"That was the understatement of all time. It was the most degrading, foul, perverted film I'd ever seen. It made me feel dirty watching it.

"I said so to Mick and he just said, 'I knew *you* wouldn't enjoy it.' We had an argument about people who get their kicks from porn, which ended in me stomping off to bed alone and him staying glued to the video."

They avoided the subject after that but Libby became obsessed with the idea that Mick had turned to porn because he was no longer turned on by her.

"When he made love to me I kept thinking of the stomach-churning things people did in that film and it would put me off. I couldn't bear to think Mick was fantasising about that filth while loving me. I felt I didn't really know him, he'd become a beast in my bed.

"It got so bad Mick could tell I was freezing when he came near me and it made him sulk and get angry. Sex was becoming more and more out of the question and Mick started going out with his mates at night and coming home drunk, something he'd rarely done all the time I'd known him.

"I thought maybe this was a dark side of him I didn't know about and seriously felt the marriage was in danger. There didn't seem any point any more."

A friend suggested counselling and initially Libby saw a counsellor on her own.

"It was very helpful. I saw how I'd shut Mick out without giving him a chance to talk about his feelings or explain anything. I learned that plenty of normal healthy young men enjoy pornographic films and magazines but it doesn't mean they're perverse. I'd come from a very straight background where things like that were thought too nasty even to talk about—normal people wouldn't watch filthy movies. Now I know they would.

"It was difficult, getting to talk things through with Mick at first because things had got so bad between us. But he agreed to come to a counselling session which helped enormously. It was less fraught talking in that calm atmosphere about things we'd never discussed.

"Afterwards, when we walked to the car holding hands for the first time in ages, I knew we'd be able to sort things out in the end. Realising how much we still loved each other was the most important step in mending our relationship."

PROBLEM: After Belinda and Chris had been married about three years, she started feeling forced into sex, a victim of her husband's voracious sex drive.

"In the beginning it was wonderful. We were at it all over the place. But after a while it started to wear me out. I'd think, 'Oh no, will he never leave me alone.' It was the relentless way he was *always* on for sex, morning, noon and night.

"If I ever looked even slightly doubtful he'd say, 'Come on, you know you'll love it.' And I couldn't possibly tell him, 'Not this time, I won't.'

"I felt like someone who'd worked in a chocolate factory and couldn't face chocolate ever again. I felt I'd had my lifetime's share of sex in three years," said 27-year-old Belinda.

She started trying to avoid it, using every excuse possible. Chris was not impressed.

"He'd never let me say no without a battle. Then we'd have a row and not speak for hours. The final straw was when he accused me of having an affair with my boss."

Belinda was so upset she went to see her doctor about her loss of interest in sex. "He said the trouble seemed to be a difference in sexual appetite and perhaps we needed some specialist help to learn how to deal with it.

"We ended up with a therapist who got us talking about our needs and feelings and who got us adapting to each other's sexual speed. The idea was that I shouldn't feel pressured by him so that he didn't then feel rejected by me.

"In the beginning, we were told to just cuddle without proceeding to sex. We had to do that for a week, which must have been hell for Chris. Then we moved on gradually till we had sex again—very differently to how it was before.

"The slow build-up made it exciting again, for both of us. Thinking about each other put a different slant on sex—it seemed more meaningful than the frantic tussles of the past. Things got better from then on."

"I'd always wanted to see her in some really raunchy gear with her high heels and stockings because I reckoned she'd look fantastic. "

PROBLEM: Alex wanted to put more excitement into bedtime, so he treated wife Kate to a saucy black lace basque and suspender belt—which she tried on once, muttered something about showing her bulges, then put away, never to be seen again.

Electrician Alex, 36, said: "I'd always wanted to see her in some really raunchy gear with her high heels and stockings because I reckoned she'd look fantastic. She didn't go in for that kind of thing, so I thought it would be a really great present to give her as a surprise.

"I said I hoped she'd do a show for me, dance around like a stripper and let me play with her suspenders and help her off with her stockings.

"I thought she'd at least give it a try, even if she thought it was nothing but a big laugh. But she didn't see the funny side, let alone want to give me a thrill in her frillies.

"She just seemed embarrassed so I thought I'd better forget it."

Alex was disappointed but couldn't think how to approach

the subject again—till he and Kate were watching a film on TV one night and one of the characters, a sexy older woman, was seducing a much younger man.

"She started peeling off her clothes, down to her bra and French knickers—and it wasn't just the young bloke who started to have breathing problems. I put my hand on Kate's knee, then I leaned over and kissed her. I said, 'You'd look even better than her, in my opinion.

"She didn't say anything then, but later, when we were getting ready for bed she said, 'Shut your eyes and count to twenty.'

"When I looked, she was standing at the end of the bed with a wicked smile, licking her lips. She was in the black lace stuff and she looked magic.

"I couldn't believe what I was seeing, at last. And she seemed to be enjoying herself. She was really out to tease me and wouldn't let me get my hands on her straight away.

"But when we finally had sex it was the most exciting ever. The best thing was she definitely threw herself into it, no holds barred. I think she surprised herself.

"Our sex life has been on the upturn ever since."

PROBLEM: Storeman Don, 35, had always made uninhibited love to girlfriend Cheryl, 30, a divorced mother of two, during passionate nights at his place.

But when she finally agreed that he should move in with her, their love life was never the same.

"She was worried about the kids and how they'd react to another man replacing their dad. That's why we waited before rushing to live together.

"I used to visit a lot and took the kids on outings with Cheryl but I never stayed the night and we tried not to kiss and hug in front of them too much.

"We all got on famously so when we told the kids I was coming to live with them,

they seemed to take it in their stride. But what we hadn't reckoned on was bedtime.

"The kids were used to popping into Cheryl's bed whenever they felt like it in the middle of the night. She'd never stopped them—why would she, when she was alone?

"So suddenly I was there and they started playing merry hell. They insisted on coming in like before. And if we tried to stop them or locked the door they threw hysterics.

"I said she had to be tough with them but she couldn't seem to do it. She always gave in, in the end.

"Sex was impossible and we started rowing over every little thing. Finally I said I'd move out because if the children were going to come between us it was hopeless.

"But luckily a friend recommended counselling to help us do the best for the children as well as ourselves. We learned how to be firm with the kids while still letting them know they were specially loved.

"Things calmed down. Now Cheryl and I are back to getting a good night's loving without interruption."

PROBLEM: Lee, a 26-year-old estate agent, had been married to wife Becky, 25, for four years. But when she wanted to start a family, he was reluctant.

"I longed for a baby so much it hurt to think about it," said Becky. "I felt the time was right. But Lee was worried about me giving up work in the recession when things weren't too good in his business.

"He said, 'Okay, if that's what you want' but I felt his fears and doubts getting in the way."

Every month she prayed to be pregnant. But when there was no sign of success after 12 months, Becky became very depressed.

"I was relieved," admits Lee. "But I couldn't bear to see her so unhappy. It was making us both miserable, so that sex was no longer a joy but more of a chore."

Becky told their GP of her fears that she and Lee couldn't produce. Also that she felt her husband wasn't too keen.

"He said we were both healthy young people and there was no reason to think we couldn't have children. But we were both in states of over-anxiety which would almost certainly be affecting our chances of parenthood.

"He advised us to stop trying for six months and for me to learn a relaxation technique like yoga—which would stand me in good stead when I eventually became a mum.

"It was brilliant. I feel better than ever, we've been having fantastic sex and I'm confident we'll have children one of these days—one way or another.

PROBLEM: Mechanic Sandy, 24, was over the moon when wife Jill, also 24, became pregnant. But then she began to repel his bedtime advances.

"All I wanted sometimes was to cuddle up tight and hug and kiss. But she was convinced it was only sex I wanted and started pushing me away, so I felt like some kind of beast," he said.

"I knew it was safe to have sex during pregnancy so I thought she was just being difficult and moody."

For the first time in his three year marriage, he found himself looking at other

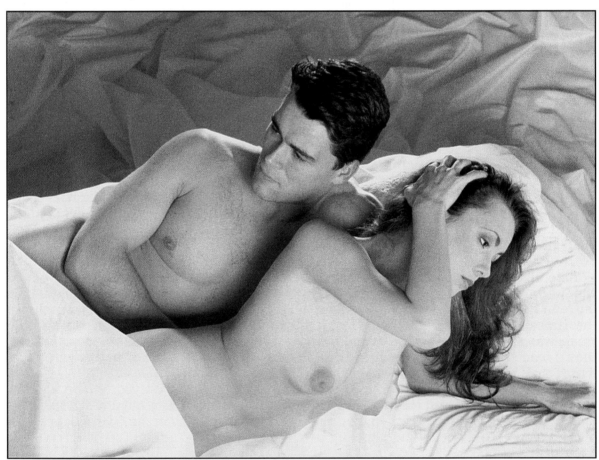

"She was convinced it was only sex I wanted and started pushing me away, so I felt like some kind of beast."

women—specially an older divorced woman with whom he worked.

"I always liked her because she was a laugh but then I realised I couldn't take my eyes or my mind off her. I was shocked to find I really fancied going to bed with her.

"One Friday night a group of us went out for a drink and it only took a few lagers to get brave. She gave me a lift home—except we stopped off at her place and things got a bit out of hand and we ended up having sex on the living room floor.

"Afterwards I felt terrible. Guilty and embarrassed. I started telling the woman I was sorry, I really loved my wife—I was confused and in a state.

"She was fantastic, considering. She told me to go home and look after Jill. She said lots of women go right off sex in the first three months—but then they often get randier than ever. So I should be patient.

"I felt a prat—but lucky I'd been saved from myself. I sent my wife AND my workmate flowers next day.

"And it was right about the sex. Jill got quite insatiable during the middle of the pregnancy—which gave us both a lot of pleasure."

PROBLEM: When sports shop assistant Gary, 22, found himself unable to rise to the occasion and satisfy Lisa, 21, his first really serious love, he was distraught.

"I never thought it could happen to me. I've had loads of girlfriends and sex was always pretty fantastic, specially with Lisa.

"When we started going out, we were at it all the time, sometimes three times a night at my flat.

"But then I moved back with my parents so I could save money. And that's when we started having problems.

"First I found I couldn't hold back in bed till Lisa was ready—we'd just get going and then it would be over in seconds, leaving her unsatisfied. Then I got so uptight I

didn't even get that far—I'd get excited all right but when we got down to business, I'd just shrivel.

"I couldn't believe I was impotent but I was so worried and scared of losing Lisa, even though she was really sympathetic. She kept saying maybe we should not try to have sex for a bit, maybe I was overtired or worried.

"But I just had to do something about it so I went to my GP to see if I had something really wrong.

"He tested me for various things and asked about my boozing habits—no problems there, I've never been a drinker. Then he asked how easy it was making love to my girlfriend in my parents' house and I had to admit it always made me feel edgy.

"They never said anything but I just felt embarrassed about it and it certainly cramped our style."

Gary's doctor guessed what the trouble was and recommended the couple go away for a weekend, somewhere they could make love from morning till night without fear of his mum walking in.

"It was amazing. We found a lovely country hotel and spent most of the weekend in bed with the Do Not Disturb sign on the door. I found no difficulty satisfying Lisa, over and over. What a relief!

"Now we go away, even for just a night, every weekend. And we're looking for a flat to share."

PROBLEM: Matt and Denise had always been ready for a randy romp and would have rated their sex life excellent—till he started taking so long to reach orgasm that Denise got not only sore but fed up.

"I'd be well satisfied but he'd be banging on for what seemed like hours and sometimes not manage a climax at all. It was frustrating for Matt and exhausting for me," said receptionist Denise, 41.

When they talked about it together, Matt

told Denise he felt that they'd got jaded and weren't trying hard enough to stimulate each other's desires.

She said: "He was right. I knew he'd always want me, even if I was wearing a potato sack. So I'd stopped trying to turn him on by looking good all the time.

"And he wasn't making much effort, either. He didn't bother shaving at weekends or washing his hair often enough.

"We suddenly looked at each other and saw we were taking each other for granted.

Sex had lost its fizz and gone decidedly flat."

They didn't need to be told what to do.

"I went to the hairdresser and had the works done, including leg waxing, manicure, pedicure. Then that night I made Matt's favourite meal, put on the soft music, lit the candles, wore my best low-cut red dress.

"He came home with red roses and a bottle of wine, had a shower and splashed on the after-shave. We had the most romantic evening in years—and Matt didn't need much urging to make full and satisfying love.

"We promised each other then that we'd never let ourselves go downhill again."

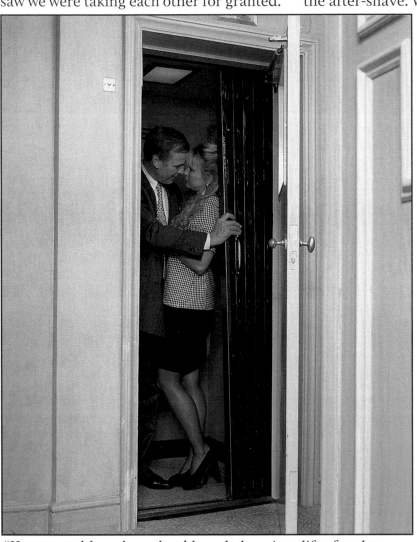

"He once told me how they'd made love in a lift after he managed to jam it between floors."

PROBLEM: Salesman Bob, 31, had had a wild affair which ended with him being dumped. When he first met 28-year-old Angie he was recovering from a broken heart and she'd helped mend it. But the shadow of the woman who hurt him kept haunting Angie.

"He once told me how they'd made love in a lift after he managed to jam it between floors. And how they did it behind the curtains in a stately home they visited.

"She had been outrageous and he was bewitched. I felt I could never excite him that much," Angie said.

"Whenever we made love and I saw his eyes closed, I always thought he was wishing it was her in his arms, not me.

"He was kind and caring and couldn't have been a better husband but I just got convinced he didn't love me.

"I started eating for comfort and soon put on two stone which made things worse. I felt unwanted and unattractive and couldn't bear him to see me undressed.

"I even insisted on making love with the lights out."

Bob could see his wife was unhappy but couldn't understand why.

"There was no reason I could think of," he said. "We had no big worries and I certainly had no interest in other women.

"I wondered if there was something I was doing to make her miserable so I thought I'd better find out."

He waited for the right moment then asked as gently as he could what was troubling Angie.

"She didn't want to talk but then it all came tumbling out, amid floods of tears.

"The funny thing was; I loved her new curvy shape—she'd always been a bit on the thin side before."

By tender loving and erotic massage of Angie's now-voluptuous body, Bob finally convinced her she was his only love.

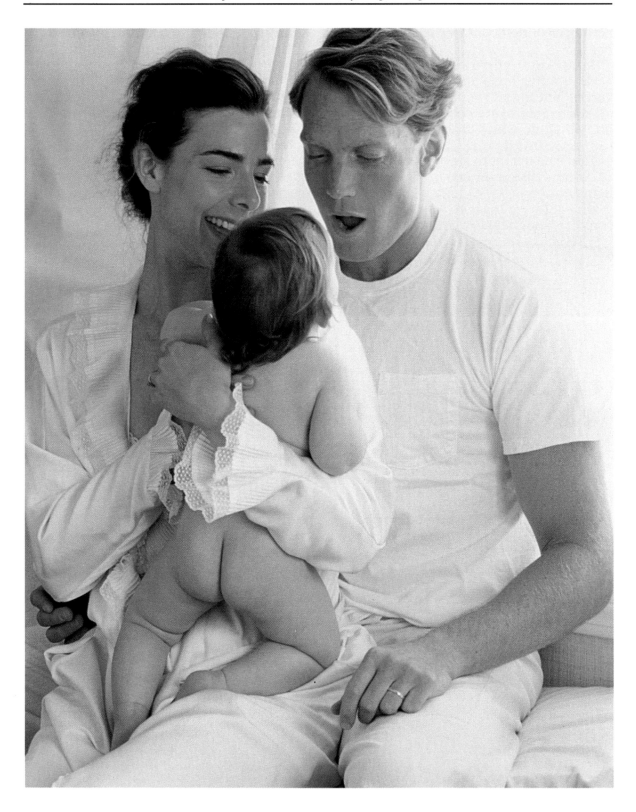

WHEN KIDS ARRIVE
Is there sex after parenthood?

You're over the moon, crazy with joy. It's confirmed and you can tell the world: we're going to have a baby. Parenthood happens to most of us sooner or later, being the natural outcome of sex. And, especially when it's the first time, we're full of wonder over what it will *really* be like.

Looking at each other, you realise with what might be a shock that very soon you'll turn from a carefree, fun-loving, sexy couple into Mum and Dad. The late nights, the parties, the boozing with mates, the dancing till dawn, the spur-of-the-moment weekend escapes—all the irresponsible pleasures of being young (or youngish) lovers with no ties are about to end.

Yes, since you ask, parenthood is certainly the end of life as you know it. But that's not to say you can't go on having fun—it's just a different kind of fun. You will know about the sleepless nights, since every parent you know will take pleasure in describing that aspect in all its mind-numbing horror. You may be shocked by the 24-hour nature of the job and the fact you can't ask babies to wait for attention nor, unless you're a heartless monster, can you ignore their cries.

What all that will do to your sex life, you can only begin to imagine at this stage. But you've no doubt heard rumours that parenthood won't boost your bonking rate.

Believe them! However, the period of zombie-like tiredness doesn't last a lifetime—and it is possible to make love when you're half asleep.

But first things first: is sex wise, possible, advisable, pleasurable, out of the question or business-as-usual during pregnancy? This is a worry for a lot of first-time parents, mainly because of the myths and scare stories of what can happen to an unborn baby if the mother indulges in a bit of nookie.

The truth is that sex during pregnancy is possible, pleasurable and shouldn't do any harm at all unless the mother-to-be has had a history of miscarriage or been told by her doctor that, for some reason, sex would be a bad idea.

On the other hand, *he* or *she* might find the thought of sex embarrassing or unappetising at this time. Some women feel so blobby and awkward about their big tums and swollen breasts that they believe even the man who loves them wouldn't want a close sexual encounter with them. This may or may not be so: most men are rather turned on by pregnant women, a pleasant surprise if you go to a party in this state and find yourself a centre of male attention. But there are some who find the idea off-putting and if your man is one of these you'll probably just have to bear with him.

Fear of harming the baby during vigorous sex is only natural. If you're fit and healthy with no known problems, your fears are probably groundless, presuming that no pregnant woman will have the agility or inclination for swing-from-the-chandeliers sex. Having an orgasm is not going to shake the unborn baby from its moorings, though the womb will have contractions like it does during labour.

The other common worry is that the penis will prod the baby and hurt it in some way. This is virtually impossible, since the penis is not a sharp object—it is, remember, made of muscle not bone and is quite small.

One of the main difficulties of sex during pregnancy is lack of desire due to hormone changes, usually in the early stages when the mother often has spells of queasiness as well. In the last three months, also, some women find their interest in sex drops close to zero. But during the middle three months, many women are actually randier than usual due, again, to rampaging hormones.

The other obvious difficulty is choosing a position that's comfortable for everyone: some men as well as women suffer discomfort and pain at this time from trying to manoeuvre themselves during intercourse.
• The sideways, or spoons, position (her back to him), is very comfortable and puts no pressure on her tum. That is why other rear-entry positions are also preferable, specially later in the pregnancy when the missionary position is not a good idea.
• Her on top; her sitting on his lap; her lying on her back with legs slung over his hips as he lies on his side facing her—all are easy positions for sex during pregnancy.
• It is better if his whole weight does not rest on her body or put pressure on her tum.
• He shouldn't thrust too fiercely but take it a bit more gently than usual.

• Her breasts will be tender to the touch and possibly sore at times, so he should treat them with tender loving care.
• If she has pains in her tum or vagina at any time, steer clear of sex
• Contractions in the womb after sex are normal and harmless and will gradually go away if she lies back in a relaxed way and lets them take their course.
• Lovemaking gives the pelvic muscles a good workout which is helpful for keeping them in good shape. After they've been stretched by the actual birth, they will get their strength and elasticity back quicker if they were well-toned beforehand.
• Use pillows to support your back, your tum, your legs or anywhere that helps you into a more comfortable position to enjoy sex.
• If you find penetrative sex too awkward, too worrying or in any way uncomfortable, why not give each other pleasure with mouths and hands?
• Unless your doctor warns otherwise, there is no reason why you shouldn't make love right up to the time you go into labour.

Once the baby has safely arrived, deciding when to resume your sex life can be tricky—once again you will hear the myths, legends and odd horror stories.

It is said to be physically safe once any bleeding has stopped and as long as the vagina feels up to it—but usually women are advised to wait six weeks.

Anyway, sex is likely to be the last thing on a woman's mind as she nurses her exhausted body, tries to stay awake to feed the new baby every four hours and perhaps is moving gingerly due to being stitched up after an episiotomy (when a cut has to be made to enable the baby's head to fit through the vaginal opening).

The new dad may be longing to wrap himself around the new mum and get passionate again without worrying about arranging their bodies so nothing is squashing anything it shouldn't. Or, if he's been present for the birth and found it all a touch traumatic as a spectator sport, he may wish to wait a while till the woman he loves gets back to her old frisky self. This is definitely a problem to discuss amongst yourselves—we all feel differently about it.

Lots of hugs, cuddles and support for each other are what's most important, never mind the timing of your first fully-fledged bonk after the event. New mums often feel flabby, stretch-marked and not their most attractive; new dads often feel neglected as new babies get all the attention from everyone, including the new mums. Having to compete for her affections with a tiny, noisy invader is more than some men can bear. So being loving, thoughtful and kind to each other is top priority over passion at this stage.

When you *do* feel the time is right to leap on each other, contraception is a must. You can't go back on the Pill till your periods return, so condoms are probably the best solution, combined with lots of lubricating jelly since new mums mostly find dryness a difficulty for a few weeks till their bodies get back to normal.

Don't be fooled into believing you can't get pregnant while breast-feeding. Most women don't ovulate while breast-feeding but some do—and you can get pregnant again after ovulating before you have your first period. Think—will you be ready to go through all this again in nine months' time? Most couples think not.

KEEPING IT FROM THE KIDS

You get through the baby stage, you've done with nappies and night feeds and nursing them to sleep. They're now toddling, talking, running, jumping livewires. They are curious, smart and everywhere. Your challenge now is how to enjoy a night, or morning, of love without them banging on the door, bursting in, or quizzing you

closely about why your bedroom door was locked. Having sex when there are kids about can be as tense as doing it on your parents' sofa as a teenager. Besides, there is no such thing as a lie-in any more or a Sunday afternoon of ravishing after the family roast. You are Mum and Dad and as far as the kids are concerned you are available every waking moment—and even if they have heard a rumour or two about sex they'll never think you two are daft, soppy or young enough to Do It.

Waiting for them to be asleep before you tentatively reach for each other's naked bodies is one way of going about it. But there are kids who never sleep as long as they know you, too, have still got your eyes open. By the time you've made sure they have lost consciousness through total exhaustion, you will be too whacked for anything more strenuous than a good night kiss.

Working out a strategy for distracting them is a better bet. Their favourite TV programme, for instance. If it's at 5 o'clock on a Saturday afternoon, say, gear your randy thoughts towards that moment. It may seem unromantic to plan your passion sessions with such precision but if you don't, you may get into a pattern of coitus interrupted by the patter of tiny feet or pounding of tiny fists on the bedroom door. If you know you can rely on 30 minutes of uninterrupted nookie-time, you can make the most of it.

Some parents don't believe in locking the bedroom door but you have to decide whether you prefer the danger element of knowing children may barge in on your lovemaking at any moment and suffer some kind of trauma from it—or the unease of knowing they are hanging about, whispering amongst themselves and perhaps setting the kitchen on fire or drowning the cat during activities to fill in time while you're at it. This is a matter of nerves and personal preference.

The one room you can lock is the bathroom. Liz, a 39-year-old mother of six, finds it the only safe haven for sex: "We do it in the bathroom all the time, even though it's incredibly uncomfortable. At least it's private. But it's not exactly warm and romantic—the floor's covered in lino and though we've endlessly tried it standing up in the shower, it's nearly impossible with my husband being a foot taller than me. I might just manage it if I sat in the soap dish."

Creating time when the two of you are guaranteed the free run of the house without the risk of the childrens' arrival to spoil your fun is the ideal. Willing and available grandparents who will take the children off your hands for a day, a night, a weekend or even a short holiday is a perfect solution.

Uninterrupted time alone is so precious it's worth doing everything you can to arrange. How about minding some friends' children for the odd weekend in return for them doing the same for you?

AND WHEN THE KIDS START ASKING EMBARRASSING QUESTIONS...

We're all upfront about sex in these enlightened days, we think, so when the children start asking questions, we plan to tell them the honest truth.

Where do babies come from? Mummy's tummy. No problem with that one—ask another.

What's oral sex? Er, well, oral means it's to do with your mouth—so oral sex is talking about it...

Hey dad, what's a Mars bar party? Hey son, who's been telling you about that?

When it comes down to it, lots of us are not brilliant at giving the simple, honest answer to our childrens' simple, straightforward questions. Our minds tend to jump around, wondering what and where our offspring heard about sex involving Mars bars—and how much should we tell an eight-year-old about such things?

The overwhelming evidence is that we would prefer our childrens' embarrassing questions about sex to be answered in the classroom—a 1987 survey found that 96 per cent of British parents thought their childrens' sex education should take place in school.

Yet every now and then, when some poor beleaguered teacher truthfully answers a question many parents would run a mile from, parents up and down the country start baying for their blood. Homosexuality, HIV/AIDS and contraception are all areas fraught with danger when it comes to discussing them with someone else's children.

What many parents don't realise is that the most important part of a child's sex education takes place before they ever get to school. Babies learn about love and affection from being cuddled, kissed and cosseted by their parents. If their parents are warm and demonstrative towards each other, kissing and hugging in front of them, babies think this is the way couples should relate to each other.

By three years, a child may be asking where babies come from. Between three and five is when most children want to know the basic facts of sex, such as how babies get into Mummy's tummy—and how they get out. They wonder about the difference between boys and girls and whether men can have babies too.

But they don't need a long biological description of the human reproductive process. They just need a short, simple and, above all, true answer. For small children, where babies come from is no more interesting than why honey falls off their toast or why Teddy sleeps with his eyes open.

Giving your kids the information they ask for when they're tiny makes it easy for them to ask more detailed questions as they grow older. Giving them duff answers only leads to mistrust when they learn the truth—they can only presume you lied to them or didn't know. Either way, they won't trust you to give them proper information again.

But suppose you don't know how to answer some of your kids' trickier questions? Embarrassment and the problem of knowing what words to use can get in the way. When this is the case, honesty is always your best policy—

• Say, 'Look here, I'm not sure about that one but I'll check it out and come back to you with the answer.'

• Say, 'Oh dear, I must admit I feel a bit funny talking to you about this. But here goes...'

• If you feel unable to talk about sex with your children, there are many excellent books and leaflets available which explain all, directly and simply. You can either give the written info to your children—or study it yourself for help in passing on the facts

• If you avoid any discussion of sex and the facts of growing up with your children they will get the idea it's a taboo subject and keep their worries to themselves. If they can't check with you that they've got their facts straight, they are likely to grow up believing all the myths, fantasies and playground half-truths—which may screw up their future relationships.

But, above all, the best favour you can do your children is show them what a happy, loving relationship between a man and a woman can be like.

Keep those hugs and cuddles coming so your children will grow up with loads of love and affection to share—the greatest start for a lifetime of Supersex!